DATE DUE

ACUPUNCTURE IMAGING

ACUPUNCTURE IMAGING

Perceiving the Energy Pathways of the Body

A Guide for Practitioners and their Patients

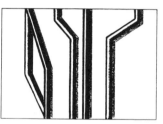

Mark D. Seem, Ph.D., Dipl.Ac. (NCCA)

Healing Arts Press
Rochester, Vermont

Healing Arts Press
One Park Street
Rochester, Vermont 05767

LIBRARY OF CONGRESS CATALOGING-IN-PUBLICATION DATA

Seem, Mark.
    Acupuncture imaging : perceiving the energy pathways of the body : a guide for practitioners and their patients / Mark Seem ; [text illustrations by William Hamilton].
      p. cm.
    Includes bibliographical references and index.
    ISBN 0-89281-375-X
    1. Acupuncture. 2. Mind and body. I. Title.
RM184.S364 1990
615.8'92--dc20   90-5066
                                                 CIP

Text illustrations by William Hamilton.

Printed and bound in the United States.

10   9   8   7   6   5   4   3   2   1

Healing Arts Press is a division of Inner Traditions International, Ltd.

Distributed to the book trade in the United States by American International Distribution Corporation (AIDC)

Distributed to the book trade in Canada by Book Center, Inc., Montreal, Quebec

Distributed to the health food trade in Canada by Alive Books, Toronto and Vancouver

Table of Contents

Acknowledgments

I would like to thank several people for their part in the production of this text:

Rosa N. Schnyer, who, when a third-year student, challenged me to articulate my style and to speak in my own name;

Fay Jean Knell, a colleague who was ever-supportive of my efforts;

Kiiko Matsumoto, whose teachings gave me the impetus to speak out for an American form of meridian acupuncture informed by palpation;

Ted Kaptchuk, for his always stimulating insights into the history of Oriental medicine as it relates to today's possibilities in this country;

June Brazil, for an excellent and patient job of word processing;

Joe Springer, for his thoughtful and probing comments.

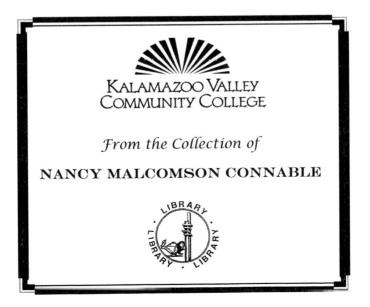

Foreword

Acupuncture Imaging, a book about Mark Seem's style of acupuncture, is more than just a record of one practitioner's idiosyncracies. In ten years of developing this style of acupuncture, Dr. Seem has thought deeply about and commented on many of the most important questions raised by American acupuncturists.

Dr. Seem here describes his own education, which resembles that of many of us who began practicing more than a decade ago. Like so many others, Dr. Seem came to acupuncture after receiving a Western education in the humanities rather than the medical sciences, and before most of the acupuncture and Chinese medical texts emanating from the People's Republic of China were available in the United States. He first studied the works of the French and Vietnamese acupuncturists, such as Soulie de Morant, Chamfrault, Schatz, Larre, and Nguyen Van Nghi, and was also influenced by Leamington acupuncture as developed by J. R. Worsley in England.

By 1983, two books had revolutionized American acupuncture. *Essentials of Chinese Acupuncture,* published in the People's Republic of China, was a basic primer written in English specifically for foreign students at the three main Chinese acupuncture schools in the People's Republic: the Beijing, Nanjing, and Shanghai Colleges of Traditional Chinese Medicine. *The Web That Has No Weaver* was an introduction to Chinese medical theory by Ted Kaptchuk, an American graduate of a Chinese medical school in Macau whose teaching was based on the curriculum in those same Chinese medical colleges.

Both of these books introduced Traditional Chinese Medicine, or TCM, to American practitioners. Although Traditional Chinese Medicine may sound like a general term covering all of Chinese medicine, as it has come to be understood in the West, it refers to a specific style of Chinese medicine developed and taught in the People's Republic of China over the last forty years. That TCM is a style of Chinese medicine rather than its totality has been amply demonstrated by such authors as Paul Unschuld, Ralph Crozier, Bruce Holbrook, Nathan Sivin, Ted Kaptchuk, and myself. Even though it is the dominant, orthodox style of Chinese medicine in China today, that fact is sometimes obscured, since contemporary Chinese sources make reference only to TCM.

At the TCM colleges in China, a new style of acupuncture was developed, and was literally called New Acupuncture in such texts as *The Barefoot Doctor's Manual* and *The Treatment of 100 Diseases by New Acupuncture.* It's methodology is based on diagnosis by discrimination of patterns of disharmony, or *Bian Zheng,* and the erection of treatment protocols mimicking the writing of a herbal prescription. Chinese herbal medicine primarily addresses itself to the Five *Zang* and somewhat less to the Six *Fu.* Therefore, it is no wonder that such a style of herbalized acupuncture is content to utilize only the Twelve Regular Channels *(Shi Er Zheng Jing)* most directly connecting to these Organs and Bowels. To these are added the *Ren* and *Du* on the sagittal midline, front and back, which in TCM acupuncture are primarily employed on the basis of their point's anatomical proximity to these Organs and Bowels. The other fifty-seven of the seventy-one Channels and Collaterals described in classical Chinese acupuncture are given little or no attention in TCM acupuncture texts.

TCM acupuncture methodology as developed in China is predicated on thrice-weekly treatments repeated over several or many weeks. When treatments are administered on such a schedule, they are relatively effective. However, because of differences in healthcare delivery in the United States, few patients can afford the time or money to receive three treatments a week for so many weeks, and without such repetitive treatment, it is questionable how effective this TCM acupuncture really is.

Like Dr. Seem, I began my acupuncture education before TCM was established as the dominant sytle here in the United States. I first studied macrobiotics and shiatsu and then learned Five Element deagnosis *a la* Worsley's Leamington Acupuncture. After that, I studied in Denver with Dr. Tao Xi-yu, who was trained in a pre-TCM, family style of acupuncture. Dr. Tao was an associate of Dr. Wu Wei-ping of Taiwan, and therefore I was also influenced by Dr. Wu's Five Element methodology. (In turn, Taiwanese acupuncture has been greatly influenced during the last ninety years by Japanese acupuncture, since, from the turn of the century until after the Second World War, Taiwan was a Japanese colony.) Concurrently, I studied French and Vietnamese acupuncture through the home-study materials prepared by the Occidental Institute of Chinese Studies. Mixed into this were also some teachings and techniques of Dr. (James) So Tin-yau, another pre-TCM Chinese acupuncturist, who had been trained in the lineage of the famous Cheng Tan-an.

When *Essentials of Chinese Acupuncture* first came out, it both excited and confused me. I was excited by the rationality and clarity of the TCM system of acupuncture, which synchronized perfectly with the Chinese herbal medicine I was already studying. However, the book also cast doubt on a great deal of what I had learned about acupunture. I therefore went to China to study at the Shanghai College of Traditional Chinese Medicine, thinking to learn from the source.

Since 1983, when I first studied at the Shanghai College, I have gained not a little insight and skill in TCM. However, I have never been impressed by TCM acupuncture, which has never worked all that well for me in the United States. It's treatments often seem close, but not quite on the mark. Patients typically respond initially but then quickly plateau. This has caused consternation both for me as a clinician and for my patients.

TCM acupuncture is a *tour de force*—an attempt to do acupuncture as if there were no substantial differences in mechanism between it and Chinese herbal medicine. Although these two Chinese healing arts are related, they are not identical, and the method of one is not entirely appropriate to the other. There are obvious mechanical differences between catalyzing healing through the ingestion of substances, and the insertion of needles through the skin.

In my experience, when acupuncture is based on classical Chinese and Japanese theories and techniques similar to those described in this book, it often acheives startlingly good results in only a few treatments, compared with the so-so results of numerous, repetitive TCM treatments. I believe this is due to the far greater precision of such acupuncture. Treatments based on these theories of Qi circulation make specific use of what acupuncture does best—the regulation of the flow of Qi. Since this Qi flows over not less than seventy-one distinct, named pathways, any one of which may be disordered, addressing consciously only fourteen of the seventy-one is bound to gloss over many patients' personal, meridian-based patterns of disharmony.

I believe that acupuncture practiced as described in *Acupuncture Imaging* is not only an acupuncturist's acupuncture but also a superior acupuncture. Dr. Seem's methodology makes natural and full use of the specific characteristics of acupuncture. Its diagnosis is primarily based on Channel and Collateral patterns of disharmony. Its diagnostic technique emphasizes palpation of the Channels and Collaterals and not just the *Cun Kou* (radial artery pulses). Its treatments address specifically those points where Qi is demonstrably, palpably blocked or deficient. In other words, this form of acupuncture is organically synchronized with its content, and more adequately meets our patient population's needs.

American patients can usually afford to come only once a week for treatment, but they look for quick results. If those results are not forthcoming, they tend to move on quickly to other therapies and therapists, since there is no lack of competing modalities in the American healthcare marketplace. At the same time, and somewhat paradoxically, our patients expect a higher level of care than that dispensed by most state-run, Chinese clinics, where the emphasis is on symptomatic relief and getting people back to work. Also, our patients are more aware of, and concerned with, their own psychology. This is not just my opinion but also the opinion of Chinese doctors who now work in the United States. As a society, we are much more sensitive to our emotions than most Chinese. Dr. Seem's style of acupuncture addresses this concern with emotional states in a way which empowers and educates his patients.

Although some TCM practitioners may think Dr. Seem unduly critical of TCM, many of his ideas and opinions are contemporary expressions of perennial themes in Chinese medicine. Dr. Seem, like the authors of the *Nei Jing* and Sun Si-miao, believes in minimal intervention. Also like Sun Si-miao of the T'ang, he sees the best role of the practitioner as an educator as opposed to a manipulator. And, like Zhang Yuan-su of the Yuan, Dr. Seem is aware that new times and places require new formulations. He is not afraid to honestly and openly search for new acupuncture forms that best fit our contemporary patients' needs and environment. It is not particularly surprising that the forms he has developed are, in fact, a return to classical acupuncture, validated by both his own experience and the best in modern science and psychology.

It is my great pleasure to recommend that American acupuncturists of all styles read *Acupuncture Imaging,* by my good friend Mark Seem. In my opinion, this book is an important contribution to the development of a uniquely American style of acupuncture and to a truly comprehensive, holistic new medicine for the twenty-first century.

Bob Flaws
Boulder, Colorado

PART I

Introduction

1

Toward Plurality in American Acupuncture

BODYMIND ENERGETICS AND ACUPUNCTURE THERAPY

During the development of the bodymind-energetic approach to acupuncture,[1] it became evident to me that I was as much educator as therapist and that I needed to articulate and execute this educational part of my work more effectively. I wished for ready access to the various pieces of information used in my work, such as the classic psychosomatic texts where clients might see their own disorders mirrored; the modern behavioral literature on the stress response, so strikingly similar to the acupuncture patterns of "Liver invading the Spleen" and "constrained Liver Qi"; diagrams of the Greater Meridian Units (Taiyin, Yangming, etc.) and the somatic-energetic reaction patterns at work in each, akin to Requena's temperaments; a survey of the basic concepts of classical acupuncture in an easily accessible fashion. I wanted, in brief, to be able to give my clients and my students a way of seeing the various elements of the phenomenological approach I had developed, drawing on ancient Eastern acupuncture energetics and modern Western psychosomatics, all in one place. I wrote *Bodymind Energetics: Toward a Dynamic Model of Health,*[2] in part as a response to this need.

After completing it, I soon realized I had to clarify in more specific terms how the new bodymind-energetic approach to acupuncture therapy translated into practice. I have written the present text to clarify, for acupuncture students and therapists interested in bodymind energetics, one possible style of acupuncture practice from this perspective.

In my way of working, still very much in process, I have come to appreciate the concept of *reframing,* as first articulated by Milton Erickson, a noted hypnotherapist. I realized that American acupuncture therapists, for example, are always engaged in reframing, or imaging their clients' disorders and complaints in the terms of acupuncture energetics and Oriental medicine, and that it was crucial to be clear about the terms in which this imaging was being carried out. I was drawing my clients into a world of somatic energetics and bodymind interrelatedness, informed by an energetic story of my own making. If they were to make real progress in our work together, I had to be clear with them about the subject of this story, namely, the *body energetic,* so that they might enter into an exploration with me that enabled them to go on to construct an energetic story of their own.

This lead me to ponder my own position, as an acupuncture therapist trained in Western philosophy and grounded in Western psychosomatics. Was I no longer an acupuncturist if I worked from such a perspective? Was I working at odds with the essence of Oriental Medicine as first articulated over two thousand years ago in China? Was the modern, Traditional Chinese Medicine approach to acupuncture, so predominant in America for the past decade, the only way to conceive of American acupuncture theory and practice, or were other ways of working also viable and in line with the ancient teachings? These were questions that came up as I set out on my own way, and it is a premise of *Bodymind Energetics* and the present text that American acupuncturists really have no choice but to develop a personal style. Obviously, if this is the case, it is best to be clear about one's own style, and what follows is one attempt in the direction of such clarity.

NEW MEDICINE AND OLD MEDICINE IN CHINA

At no time in its long history, except for a short 30-year period perhaps already coming to a close, has Chinese Medicine developed "a coherent and—in a western sense—consistent—set of ideas and patterns. . . ."[3] As can already be witnessed in *The Yellow Emperor's Classic of Internal Medicine,* according to Paul Unschuld, a University of Munich expert in Chinese medical history, a characteristic trait in the history of Chinese medical thought is that antagonistic concepts within a major paradigm—such as Yin Yang or the Five Phases—were rarely resolved in the development of a synthesis of the two. No single paradigm, therefore, ever achieved dominance. What is characteristic of the Chinese medical tradition, therefore, is a "continuous tendency toward a syncretism of all ideas that exist. . . . Somehow a way was always found in China to reconcile opposing views and to build bridges—fragile as they may appear to the outside observer—permitting thinkers and practitioners to employ liberally all the concepts available."[4] Rather than a unified system of thought and practices, there existed a "collection of the teachings of numerous schools of various times," even as early as the *Yellow Emperor's Classic.*[5]

Less than three decades ago, in accordance with Mao's famous mandate to uncover and upgrade the treasures of traditional Chinese medicine, the first effort was made to establish a unified system, to be the "New Medicine" of China.[6] In the texts written or translated for a Western readership, the

Oriental medicine aspect of this new medicine was labeled "Traditional Chinese Medicine" (TCM). The label is inappropriate for two reasons. First, it obscures the fact that there has never been one traditional medicine of China. Second, it misleads many students into thinking that this very modern reformulation of Chinese medicine is "traditional" when it is, in fact, a recent invention.

In the past few years the brief history of TCM has taken a turn whereby "New Medicine is no longer a central goal of healthcare planning in the People's Republic of China."[7] Rather, there is a movement afoot more consistent with the long history of Chinese medicine, toward a plurality of therapeutic principles and practices that perhaps accounts in part for the renewed interest in traditional practices such as Qi Gong (breath control exercises) that fell out of favor during the Cultural Revolution.

It would therefore be anachronistic in terms of the modern developments in Chinese medicine, and ahistorical in the broader sense, for Western practitioners and teachers of acupuncture and Chinese medicine to remain wed to the illusion of one, "true" Traditional Chinese Medicine.

The TCM style of acupuncture has dominated the American scene for the past several years, mainly because the key texts available in the West date from the era of the "New Medicine," and many American acupuncture educators were trained in this style either in schools here or in China. This situation is beginning to change as texts appear that stem from other traditions of acupuncture. These include the Japanese styles surveyed by Kiiko Matsumoto, the French and English styles articulated in Royston Low's study of meridian energetics and Yves Requena's own constitutional theory, and the work of various American practitioners trained in pre-TCM styles of acupuncture therapy.[8]

What was once a rigid, almost dogmatic tendency of American acupuncture to adhere to the tenets of TCM as the only true acupuncture is giving way to a growing curiosity about other traditions and styles of acupuncture and Oriental medicine.

In America, then, we have the opportunity to participate in the reformulation of Oriental medicine to meet our own specific intellectual and healthcare needs. What emerges as American acupuncture will necessarily be different from what is being practiced elsewhere, and it will reflect the plurality of traditions and schools of thought that inform American practices and teachings.

This sort of foreign influence on the development of Chinese medicine is not new, as Unschuld informs us regarding the late Chou dynasty in China, where innovative medical doctrines formulated by Chinese thinkers quite possibly included assimilation of outside concepts and practices. There is nothing surprising about this in the history of medical thought, Unschuld emphasizes, for foreign influences are always translated and reformulated to meet local conditions, in a discourse reflecting the mode of medical thought of those who assimilate the foreign ideas. Unlike the travel of merchandise, where one could easily trace the transportation of goods from a foreign culture to ones own, the travel of ideas is different: "Ideas must be transmitted by the head, and, of necessity, will undergo change. Where could a foreign idea be accepted, assimilated, or transmitted without being influenced by the particular situation it meets, by the changing languages that serve as its means of transportation, and by the preconditioned patterns of thought cherished by the final receiver?"[9]

The present text is written in that same spirit of transmission and transformation. The goal in the following pages is to present one style of practice, stemming from French, TCM, and Japanese influences, and informed by a Western psycho-somatic and behavioral perspective. The philosophical under-pinnings for this bodymind-energetic[10] approach to acupunc-ture have been developed in *Bodymind Energetics,* and the current attempt is toward clarification of the personal style developed over a ten-year period that stems from this perspec-tive as it relates to the practice of acupuncture in this country.

2

A Question of Style

In articulating my own ongoing development of a style, I am not attempting to forge a new school of thought. Rather, I am voicing, in my own name, my efforts at the establishment of a *teaching* at the Tri-State Institute of Traditional Chinese Acupuncture, which I direct, based on the premise that all students and practitioners of American acupuncture must work to clarify their own styles, and learn ultimately to speak in their own names, rather than mimic the teachings of their teachers.

In an exercise with various student and faculty groups at our institute, all had to share their clinical priorities on a given pattern or case, stating which diagnostic criteria they would opt for. What was clear in this exercise was that certain people resorted first to the rubric of "Qi, Blood, Fluids" to filter the clinical data in order to arrive at a diagnosis, while others resorted more readily to the rubric of the "Patterns of Disharmony," and so forth. It was apparent to me that I did not select the same filters as many of my students and faculty, or selected them in an entirely different order of preference. This was pointed out by a student-intern in a clinic session early in her third year, who noticed that I rarely spoke of "Qi, Blood, and Fluids," for example, and only spoke of patterns within the larger context of meridian-energetic imbalance.

The current text is written for the benefit of my students, on the small scale, to clarify my way of working (in progress) and to prod them to develop their own ways over time after they graduate. It is also written in the hope that more American practitioners will open up and share, beyond their stated ideological positions (for example, as practitioners of TCM or of the Worsley School), how they really perceive the energetics of those with whom they work, and how they actually arrive at a diagnosis and treatment plan. Such sharing will reveal personal biases which, if acknowledged, can be personal strengths. If not openly noticed, they may serve as stumbling blocks or blind spots in a practitioner's future development.

In a course on Ericksonian hypnotherapy, I was struck by the concept of reframing. What was clear to me as I heard these concepts was that I practiced reframing, which I refer to as imaging in the following discussion, every time I treated a client. In each case, the client's conditions, complaints, and disturbances were reformulated in energetic terms which, when shared with the client, served as powerful new means of perceiving the bodymind imbalances that often led to a bodily felt sense (Gendlin) of the energetic nature of the imbalance. Such a sense was like an energetic sensory awareness that the client seemed to already possess on some level. Over time, I came to conceive of my work not as treatment of complaints and disturbances, but rather as a prod to enable my clients to recollect and remember the bodymind functions they had temporarily lost touch with. I no longer saw the needles as healing tools per se, but rather viewed the imaging of complaints in energetic terms as the precondition for the effectiveness of the needles once they were inserted. I began to trace the pathways carefully on the client, to help him feel the areas of conflict and to visualize how they would flow when restored to more normal functioning. Often I would ask, after inserting the needles, whether I had left a point or area untouched that needed to be touched. To my initial surprise, the client would often immediately point to a specific point or energetic zone that made perfect sense, and at times served, when needled, to move the transformation process much further or faster.

The conclusion, for me, after ten years of treating people with acupuncture therapy, was evident. I personally was not a healer, but an educator in the strict sense, guiding my clients, I hoped, to a new understanding of their bodymind energetics. The bodymind integrated perspective of acupuncture energetics, and the wonderfully detailed and complex acupuncture understanding of the *body energetic,* were my biases—my point of departure. When I shared these insights with my clients, and entered into an imaging of their complaints or situations in acupuncture bodymind-energetic terms, they were helped to gain contact with a hidden, or perhaps even lost, self-awareness of the integrative, healing capacities of the bodymind's will to be well.

I hope that as people work in this *acupuncture imaging* way, they will be helped to construct an energetic story of their complaints that serves as a starting point for movement beyond the body/mind split entailed by the complaint.

My own orientation is acupuncture energetics, not Oriental medicine, as I do not practice herbology or other forms of Chinese medicine. By *acupuncture energetics,* I mean *a practice with the intention that, in treatment of a pattern of points, they resonate with archaic pathways of the bodymind.* I picture my treatments along the pathways of the meridian systems selected, and work to align my focus and the client's attention to these energetic zones. My belief is that when this is done, the client's true healing intention can be channelled to the appropriate zones, thereby affecting a bodymind integration leading to change.[1]

To me, acupuncture energetics is similar to tattooing a sign on a tribe member's face to mark him as belonging to a particular region and clan, and no other, rooting a body solidly on the soil from whence it sprang. By tracing and prodding the pathways of the body, acupuncture is primal, territorial, and brings a person into deep contact with his body, body-image, and Self. Body-image is always touched by acupuncture, for the needling intervenes in the surface space where body armoring and defenses are at play in their effort to enable an individual to retain the integrity of body, mind, and spirit in relation to the outside world. While the concept of body-image evoked here, and especially articulated in Chapter 4 of *Bodymind Energetics*, is informed by classic psychoanalytic psychosomatics, it is actually surprisingly close to the ancient acupuncture conceptualization of the organ-energetic functions, according to the renowned French sinologist and expert in Chinese medical terminology, Father Claude Larre. In his discussion of the *Hun*, the spirit of the Liver energetic function, Larre clearly articulates the ancient Chinese conception of body-image: "By hereditary coding man would have the power to call up in himself the images that would guarantee all his functions from the smallest to the most highly evolved."[2] This concept of visceral or vegetative spirit implies that acupuncture stirs an individual's memory of how these various organ-energetic spirits work in concert for bodymind integrity at all levels of the organism.

The pathways of acupuncture energetics, then, which many modern practitioners of the new TCM style of acupuncture seem to be leaving behind in favor of a mechanical use of points for their (supposedly) specific effect on a given symptom or disease, hark back to the first imprints in the mother's womb, where the code for the future functioning of the individual is laid down in its entirety. Acupuncture energetics is in the service of this code, respects the uniqueness of each individual, and works to help the person remember the nature of this code. To treat points for specific symptoms or diseases, without a larger perspective that recognizes the primal nature of the energetic pathways of acupuncture, deterritorializes a person: it separates symptom and person, object and subject, divorcing him from his own space. While the actual needling of the point is a sympathetic nervous system stimulant, catalyzing movement and change, the entire treatment process is usually one whereby the individual sinks into a parasympathetic relaxation phase for a few moments, often more profound than one is usually accustomed to. By allowing an individual to remember energetic pathways that have been forgotten or mistreated, a person is able to sink, safely and briefly, into the undifferentiated, pre–organ-functional, energetic field (body without organs, prior to body-image), where sharply defined contours forced on the bodymind by the outside world dissolve. Many clients remark on this undifferentiated feeling, as if they were not in the world but in another undefined space, where the body merged with the cosmos. This is reminiscent of the peace of being cradled in the mother's arms, itself harking back to the uterine space (called the primal embrace by some psychosomaticians). The infant sinks into its mother's arms after a day of discovery and adventure in the outside world (sympathetic system activity), exhausted from the day's activity. This parasympathetic sinking down into its undifferentiated self enables the infant to emerge the next day, or after the nap, ready for more activity, learning, and growth. In like fashion, acupuncture seems to facilitate a client's movement inward, into that same safe place, relaxed and ready to emerge better equipped for activity in the world. People emerge from treatment revitalized yet calmer (a paradox to many stressed people who think that energy means agitation), with a greater awareness of their bodymind's potential for change.

That, at least, is my way of perceiving acupuncture energetics, and the above images inform the way of working to be articulated in the following pages.

Part II

Acupuncture Influences and Styles

3

French Acupuncture Influences

HUMAN ENERGETICS

The primary influence on my style of practice comes from the various French teachings adopted by the Quebec Institute of Acupuncture, where I trained, and its main teachers, Drs. Van Nghi, Schatz, and Wexu. Further reading and translation of works by the father of French Acupuncture, George Soulie de Morant, and study and discussions with Dr. Yves Requena, enriched my perspective.

In *L'Energetique humaine*[1] Dr. Chamfrault, a pioneer of French acupuncture, and Dr. Van Nghi, a French trained physician-acupuncturist and translator and commentator on Vietnamese acupuncture works, expanded upon the human energetics of acupuncture as already described by Soulie de Morant in his major works on the subject. In this view, acupuncture brought the realm of energetics so crucial in physics into the practice of medicine. The various energetic systems, constituting meridian energetics, were therefore seen as constituting a different framework by which to understand the body and its functioning as well as its disorders. These early practitioners strove to explain in great detail the complex energetics of acupuncture, through careful reading of major classic and modern texts from China, Japan, and Vietnam.

They saw the need to experiment with the treatment strategies of classical acupuncture, rather than reinterpret these strategies into Western medical pathophysiological terms. The fact that all but Soulie de Morant were medical doctors makes it all the more impressive that these original French practitioners respected acupuncture energetics in its own right and sought to gain as much expertise as possible in its classical application. This often differs from the approach of many American physician acupuncturists, who usually train for only a few hundred hours and learn acupuncture as if it were a simple adjunct to pain control according to Western physiological parameters.

It was Van Nghi, particularly in the above-mentioned text and in his seminal *Pathogenie et Pathologie en Medecine Traditionelle Chinoise*, who provided the understanding of the surface energetics represented by the tendino-muscular, divergent, and Luo vessels, and the primal energetics of the Eight Extraordinary Vessels. Most schools of acupuncture in the United States did not teach this system of surface and deep energetics, relying instead on the texts being translated by the People's Republic of China such as *The Outline of Chinese Acupuncture* and *The Essentials of Chinese Acupuncture*. In these TCM texts, descriptions of the energetics of the secondary and extraordinary vessels were totally absent, leading many American-trained practitioners to think that the meridian system—comprising, as they thought, only fourteen pathways—was rather simple indeed. As stated in the introduction, the texts from the PRC over the past two decades have been conspicuously devoid of meridian energetics, so it is no wonder that American teachings often followed suit. Couple this with the fact that the teachings regarding the Five Elements in this country were derived from English schools, where the only translation of the *Huang-ti-nei-ching* was the unacceptable version by Ilza Veith, and where this knowledge was sometimes divorced from an understanding of the meridian-energetic system to which the Five Element teachings relate, and it is clear that the American knowledge of acupuncture energetics was greatly deficient from the time of its early development through the seventies. This is beginning to change with the translation of Japanese and French texts and owing to the fine summary of meridian energetics by Royston Low *(Secondary Vessels of Acupuncture)*.

My own practice was influenced from the start by these French meridian-energetic teachings. I was taught, almost without realizing it, to appreciate the need to regulate the upper and lower zones of the body, paying careful attention to front and back and right and left energetic polarities. For example, if I found constriction in the left leg branch of the Liver meridian, I would palpate the body's energetic zones related to Liver: palpating the right leg branch; palpating all along the pathway on the left to see if the local constriction in the leg was due to blockage of energy elsewhere along its path; checking the corresponding upper branches of Jueyin, namely the Pericardium pathway, first on the right, as right/left—upper/lower imbalances are so common (constituting, in meridian energetics, what body workers term compensation); then on the left (perhaps Jueyin is constricted on the left, and deficient on the right, for example); also paying attention to the paired meridian, the Gallbladder (perhaps the Gallbladder pathways are excess, and the Liver deficient, leading to local constriction). This attention to the various connections to the left Liver energetic zone is very similar to the palpation one observes when watching Japanese teachers, such as Kiiko Matsumoto, as they conscientiously palpate the body energetic to assess the total energetic condition of the organism. It is very different from palpating the pulses alone, which, according to the modern

TCM teachings, correlate with the ZangFu, *not* the meridians. Also, significantly, the secondary vessels (tendino-muscular, divergent, Luo) and the Eight Extraordinary Vessels do not tend to show up on the pulses. One must know their general characteristics, symptomatology, energetic zones of influence and convergence, and modes of treatment, which are totally different in principle from the treatment of the regular meridians. The Five Element principles taught by some schools, for example, do not apply to the use of the secondary vessels and Eight Extraordinary Meridians, and since the latter constitute the bulk of the energetic system of acupuncture, Five Element treatment strategies apply only seldom. The two dominant styles of practice in this country—TCM and Five Element acupuncture—both emphasize the ZangFu (called Officials by Five Element practitioners of the Worsley school) and the regular meridians only, and ignore the complex surface and primal energetic networks, which, taken as a whole with the regular meridians, constitute *human energetics*. In this sense, they are *disembodied* approaches to acupuncture.

SURFACE ENERGETICS

The reader is referred to *The Secondary Vessels of Acupuncture* by Royston Low,[2] which describes in detail the internal energetics of the regular meridians, as well as the secondary vessels and Eight Extraordinary Vessels, for the basics of the French human-energetic teachings. The appreciation gained for surface energetics, as a kind of character armoring, in reading the French teachings will raise many questions for practitioners who have limited their practice to Five Element strategies. For example, if what they actually witness in a particular case of excess of the Liver meridian is excess of the tendino-muscular aspect of this meridian system, with a relative deficiency of the deeper, regular meridian, but they treat it as an excess of the regular meridian by sedating the Liver meridian, this would allow for a penetration of the disorder, hitherto lodged solely in the tendino-muscular zone of the surface, deep into the regular meridian, now sedated and unable to withstand such a penetration. To treat virtually every disorder as if it were a deep energetic imbalance, which many Five Element-trained as well as TCM-style practitioners often do, presuming problems to be at the deep ZangFu level (since they have little concept of the surface energetics under discussion here), bypasses the surface energetic zones and perhaps allows for a weakening of this zone by treating too deeply, too often.

Japanese and French-trained practitioners seem to appreciate these surface energetic systems much more, and often treat locally and superficially (those who have trained in the PRC over the past decade must wonder whether the Chinese even know how to needle superficially, given the preponderance of very deep, very strong needling practiced by TCM practitioners of acupuncture) to free up energetic obstruction, knowing that in freeing up the surface they are tonifying deeper energetic pathways and functions. This *meridian energetic intention* is what constitutes the singularity of many French and Japanese styles. Practitioners with such an intention not only have an abstract idea of an organ-function or Official in which they expect to see change as a result of the treatment, but are keenly aware, first and foremost, of a precise, palpable energetic pathway or zone which they expect to see freed up, strengthened, or brought into harmony with another zone of the body energetic.

In the French teachings evoked above, the meridian-energetic system is thought to develop from the moment of conception to adulthood. First to appear are the three extraordinary meridians, Chung Mo, Ren Mo, and Du Mo. These three serve as the body energetic's chief *organizers*,[3] and each structures the energetic zones which it influences—Chung Mo energizing the front of the body and nourishing the visceral functions (it is the *potential* for ZangFu functions, the energetic basis upon which the Zang and Fu later develop); Ren Mo in relationship with Du Mo, the former constituting Yin energies and forming the ventral surface, and the latter constituting Yang energies and forming the dorsal surface. To this longitudinal energetic flow there comes a fourth meridian, Daimo, which encircles the other three, directing the activities of upper/lower parts of the body energetic. Together, these constitute the front/back and upper/lower energetic zones. The other four extraordinary meridians—Yinchiaomo, Yangchiaomo, Yinweimo, and Yangweimo—organize the particular Yin and Yang energetics of the four quadrants, connecting upper left with lower right, and vice versa.

The second set of meridians to develop is the tendino-muscular meridians, in close relationship with the Liver, which controls the free flow of musculature, connective tissue, the diaphragm (under the control of the Liver), and the serous membranes of the abdominal and thoracic regions of the body. Their function is to bar access of perverse energies to the deeper, regular meridians and ZangFu functions, and they also serve as a kind of character armoring, according to several French writers.

Next to develop are the regular meridians, followed by the Luo and divergent pathways.

While nourishing and ancestral energy travel in the extraordinary vessels, Wei defensive energy circulates in the tendino-muscular and divergent pathways, and Ying nourishing energy flows in the regular meridians and their Luo vessels.

The key, in the French meridian energetic approach (Van

Nghi especially), is to know which energetic level—defensive, nourishing, ancestral—is affected and to treat the corresponding energetic network.

In *Terrains and Pathology in Acupuncture*, Dr. Yves Requena, a physician and student of Van Nghi, expands upon the Great Meridian Units (Taiyang, Shaoyin, etc.) to develop a concept of temperaments which I have reviewed in detail in *Bodymind Energetics*. While I do not feel that it is valid to postulate strict one-to-one relationships between the scanty descriptions of those Great Units as personality types in the *Nei-Ching* and corresponding temperaments in French morphological systems, I do find it fascinating to think about the predispositions of someone with a Taiyang energetic configuration, or of someone with a Jueyin configuration, etc. American practitioners tend to develop a sense of the psychology (in the Western sense) of the acupuncture system, which needs to be further developed, and Requena's work in this direction is exemplary.

Since I find that the majority of a person's disorders develop along the pathways energized by the Great Units, Requena's categorization of pathology in terms of Taiyang, Shaoyang, Yangming, Taiyin, Jueyin, and Shaoyin is extremely useful and accurate. Someone with a predisposition to dysfunction along the Shaoyang zones of Gallbladder and Triple Warmer pathways will develop characteristic disorders in each of the systems of the body different from those of someone who is predisposed to dysfunction along the Taiyin pathways of Lung and Spleen. I take these in a behavioral way, as *somatic energetic reactivity zones*. Hence, Taiyin is a zone of reactivity entailing all of the various Spleen and Lung pathways (from tendino-muscular to regular and Luo) that can be brought into play because one has an energetic imbalance either due to heredity or early childhood events in Lung or Spleen, or due to later trauma to either of these energetic zones. In other words, as soon as Lung or Spleen are disturbed, the whole of Taiyin is predisposed to dysfunction. This type of somatic energetic reactivity is frequently what we face in acupuncture therapy, and I shall discuss one view of how to treat it presently. Whether as a *constitutional factor* or as a privileged zone of *coping mechanisms,* Taiyin would thus constitute, in this instance, a target zone whose vulnerability would recur as a major factor in all complaints experienced by this individual.

Taken as a whole, the French meridian-energetic teachings allow us to undertake more finely tuned energetic interventions to accurately prod the bodymind of our clients. If the goal of acupuncture therapy is, indeed, to guide the client to a recollection of his bodymind-energetic functioning, then the better our knowledge of energetics, the more precisely we will be able to prod our client's recollection.

MEETING ZONES

Below is a list of key meeting zones and zones of confluence of energies according to the French meridian teachings. Royston Low's excellent text contains more details.

The Three Powers (Heaven-Earth-Man)[4]

Governing Vessel (G.V.) 20 corresponds to Heaven.
Conception Vessel (C.V.) 17 corresponds to Man.
Kidney 1 corresponds to Earth.

The Three Levels of the Body[5]

Spleen 21 corresponds to chest level.
Stomach 25 corresponds to middle level.
Spleen 8 corresponds to lower level.

ROOTS AND NODES OF THE SIX MERIDIANS

The *root* is the point of polarization, where transformation from yin to yang and vice versa occurs. The *node* is the point where the great unit's energy is most concentrated.

Taiyang

> Root = Bladder 67.
> Node = Bladder 1.

Yangming

> Root = Stomach 45.
> Node = Stomach and Large Intestine meeting zone (L.I. 19–20; St. 3–4).

Shaoyang

> Root = Gallbladder 44.
> Node = area in front of ear (G.B. 1 and 3; T.H. 22 and 23).

Taiyin

> Root = Spleen 1.
> Node = C.V. 12.

Jueyin

> Root = Liver 1.
> Node = C.V. 18.

Shaoyin

> Root = Kidney 1.
> Node = C.V. 23.

TENDINO-MUSCULAR MEETING ZONES

- Three Yang tendino-muscular meridians of the Foot (St., Bl., GB.) = area from S.I. 18–St. 5
- Three Yang tendino-muscular meridians of the Hand (L.I., T.H., S.I.) = Gallbladder 13
- Three Yin tendino-muscular meridians of the Foot (Sp., Liv., Kid.) = Conception Vessel 3
- Three Yin tendino-muscular meridians of the Hand (Ht., Per., Lu.) = Gallbladder 22

UNION POINTS

- Stomach 12 = union of L.I., T.H., GB., Lu., St., S.I.
- Governing Vessel 14 = union of all Yang meridians.
- Bladder 1 = union with St., T.H., Bl., Yinchiaomo, and Yangchiaomo.
- S.I. 10 = union with Yangweimo and Yangchiaomo.
- S.I. 12 = union with S.I., L.I., T.H., G.B.
- C.V. 17 = union with T.H., Sp., Ht., Liv., Per.
- Bl. 11 = union with S.I. and T.H.

DIVERGENT MERIDIAN UNIONS

- Bladder 54 (40) = Kidney and Bladder divergent meridians meet (Shaoyin/Taiyang).
- Conception Vessel 2 = Liver and Gallbladder divergent meridians meet (Jueyin/Shaoyang).
- Stomach 30 = Stomach and Spleen divergent meridians meet (Yangming/Taiyin).
- Gallbladder 22 = Small Intestine and Heart divergent meridians meet (Taiyang /Shaoyin).

- Triple Heater 16 = Triple Heater and Pericardium divergent meridians meet (Shaoyang/Jueyin).
- Stomach 12 to Large Intestine 18 = Large Intestine and Lung divergent meridians meet (Yangming/Taiyin).
- Stomach 4 = union of Ren Mo and Chung Mo with Stomach regular meridian ("Oral Point").

MENTAL SYMPTOMS AND SIGNS

Below are lists of mental symptoms associated with disturbance of the meridians and the Organ-functions (ZangFu) according to French Sources, similar in some respects to symptoms associated with the "Officials" in Worsley's teachings.

Mental Signs of Meridian Disorders [6]

Lung. Excess: obsessions that are future directed. Deficiency: a feeling of being vulnerable.

Large Intestine. Mental confusion, defective elimination of ideas, stubbornness, complacency in being wrong, rigidity of thinking, vulnerability to the cold.

Stomach. Depression, death wishes, instability, suicidal tendencies, mentally overwrought, doubt, suspicions, tendency to mania, slowness at assimilating ideas.

Spleen. Mental sluggishness, vertigo, melancholia, obsessions turned towards the past, fixed and rigid ideas, sleepwalking, agitated sleep, nightmares.

Heart. All shen disturbances, insomnia, anxiety.

Small Intestine. Poor mental assimilation, a feeling of mental deficiency due to inability to assimilate ideas, insecurity.

Bladder. Changeable moods, over-enthusiasm, suspicion, jealousy, lack of confidence, mental lassitude.

Kidney. Anxiety, fear in the pit of the stomach, sadness, mental and physical fatigue, antisocial tendencies, laziness.

Pericardium (Heart Protector). Depression, sexual perversion, aversions, phobias.

Triple Heater. Emotional upsets caused by breaking of friendships or family relations, depression, suspicion, anxiety, poor elimination of harmful thoughts.

Gall Bladder. Bitterness, lack of control, irritability, unfaithfulness, lack of courage, timidity, hypochondria.

Liver. Irritability, difficulty developing ideas, depression, lack of energy.

Mental signs of ZangFu Disturbances [7]

Lung Zang. Excess: panting, yawning, sneezing. Deficiency: cold shoulder and back, changing complexion, inability to sleep.

Heart Zang (Pericardium essentially the same). Excess: false or facile laughter, sobbing, agitated spirit. Deficiency: sadness, absence of laughter, depression, fear, anxiety, shortness of breath.

Spleen Zang. Excess: heaviness (excess "form"), large abdomen, great sighing, sadness, obsessions, nightmares. Deficiency: slightness (deficient "form"), abundant elimination, morning fatigue, cold, wet feet.

Kidney Zang. Excess: over-decisiveness; dreams of difficulty undoing one's belt (G.V. 4 as part of Daimo); heavy, hot, painful legs. Deficiency: indecisive; confused speech; dreams of trees submerged under water; cold feet and legs; abundant sweating.

Liver Zang. Excess: discontent, anger, priapism, pain in

lumbar region and genitals. Deficiency: impotence; frigidity; pain in thighs, pelvic region, and throat; ready tendency to "the blahs."

Large Intestine Fu. Excess: dry mouth, parched lips, hot body. Deficiency: skin eruptions, itching, cold, difficulty in warming up.

Small Intestine Fu. Excess: happiness, joviality, scarlet complexion. Deficiency: bluish lips with white border, emaciation, profuse sweating.

Stomach Fu. Excess: nightmares, acne, skin eruptions, over active stomach (excess acid). Deficiency: slow digestion, vomiting after meals, painful eyebrows, emotionality, teariness, sadness, cold feet.

Bladder Fu. Excess: agitation, excessive erections, prostatitis, frequent and urgent need to defecate, headaches on defecation. Deficiency: lack of confidence, lethargy, neurological disorders, low sexual energy, incontinence.

Gallbladder Fu. Excess: tiredness, sighing, irritability, bitter taste in mouth in the morning, pain in all joints, edematous knees and legs. Deficiency: insomnia, wandering pains, chest and side pains, swollen breasts.

These mental signs figure in the more comprehensive character types of Yves Requena. The reader is referred to his text for a description of these temperamental types, and to Chapter 3 of *Bodymind Energetics* for a critical appraisal of this mixing of Chinese character sketches and French modern character typing and for a review of J. R. Worsley's depiction of the "Officials".[8] Like the English, whose early practitioners often had access to the French teachings of de Morant and Lavier in their training, the French often felt the need to expand upon the personality profiles that correspond to the organ-energetic functions and meridians.

Given that the classical acupuncture texts show no separation of mental and somatic symptoms, all of which might figure in a disorder of a particular energetic zone or unit, it is important for Western acupuncture practitioners to observe carefully that place where the psyche and the body process converge in energetic disturbances. This attention to mental as well as physical signs and symptoms allows one to hone in more accurately on a person's energetic imbalance while at the same time developing a truly client-centered acupuncture therapy that seeks to educate the client about his ways of being and coping in the world, rather than just treating him for some supposedly objective syndrome or complaint.

An appreciation of bodymind interaction and a detailed focus on the complexity of meridian energetics, with a special focus on the upper/lower Great Meridian Units, is what characterizes these French teachings, which have influenced my own style. In some ways, this is very similar to the teachings of various Japanese educators, as presented by Kiiko Matsumoto in her fine works, to be studied in the next section.

4

Some Japanese Styles: Palpating the Energetic Core[1]

In the conclusion to *Extraordinary Vessels*, Kiiko Matsumoto and Stephen Birch point a way for American acupuncture, beyond what I shall term TCM acupuncture, that brings us back to the traditional acupuncture practices focused on human energetics rather than on diseases and their treatment.

A brief digression concerning my own training in acupuncture as one example of the complicated path through which the earlier American practitioners of acupuncture had to weave their way, may clarify this discussion of the differences between core acupuncture energetics and TCM acupuncture as practiced in the West.

In my earliest acupuncture training, under practitioners and teachers schooled at the Quebec Institute of Acupuncture in Montreal, we used the *Outline of Chinese Acupuncture* as our guide to the locations of points and acupuncture techniques, but used European texts—Lawson and Woods, Austin, Mann, Van Nghi, Chamfrault, and Schatz—to guide our deeper journey through acupuncture and to base our philosophical perspective on acupuncture energetics. No one talked in those early days of Traditional Chinese Medicine (TCM—a term coined after the *Essentials of Chinese Acupuncture*), and there was scant discussion of oriental herbology. The focus was entirely on the theories and manipulation of "human energetics," a term that became the title of an important treatise on secondary vessels by Dr. Chamfrault, himself a student of Soulie de Morant, and Dr. Van Nghi, a Vietnamese physician and major translator of Vietnamese acupuncture works. The French writings by de Morant, Chamfrault, Van Nghi, and Schatz, to name the main early authors, focused on the practice of acupuncture as an energetic therapeutic approach that conceived of the human body as an energetic field of complex forces. This view brought concepts and theories strikingly similar to modern physics into the realm of Western medicine (all those authors but de Morant are physicians). Therapeutic discussion centered on the ways in which one must tend to the Roots (core energetics) while also subduing the Branches of a given complaint, and these authors were very clear that Root treatment was preventive in nature, and brought into play the Eight Extraordinary Vessels and Five Element acupuncture strategies. This is exactly the point of view of the Japanese practitioners studied by Matsumoto and Birch.

What is striking in American acupuncture about this *human energetics* perspective is that it has been all but supplanted by the TCM, herbalized acupuncture that arose in the People's Republic of China during the Cultural Revolution, which speaks little if at all of the extraordinary and secondary vessels or of the Five Element strategies, replacing them with more localized treatment strategies that focus on specific symptoms or symptom–sign complexes (syndromes). Rather than speak of "transferring energy," a term which does not appear even once in the *Essentials* or in *Acupuncture: A Comprehensive Text* (a translation of another major TCM book from the People's Republic of China, by Bensky and O'Connor), TCM acupuncture displays a decidedly "herbalized" way of combining points.

Flaws, Chace, and Helme clarify this herbalized TCM acupuncture in their book, *Timing and the Times: Chronicity in the American Practice of Oriental Medicine,*[2] thus: "Twentieth century practitioners of TCM such as Wang Le-ting have consciously and deliberately created acupuncture protocols based on famous herbal prescriptions where each point or group of points mimics the action of a specific herbal ingredient. Since many American acupuncture schools have adopted this version of acupuncture as the basis for their curriculum, this style has also gained ascendancy in America today." The authors point out that modern practitioners of TCM acupuncture in China have abandoned the ancient energetic transfer strategies in favor of combinations that have been demonstrated to be clinically effective. This fits the mandate of Mao for a modernized revival of traditional Chinese medicine beyond metaphysics, as well as the trend in the People's Republic of China during the better part of the twentieth century toward Western medicine. It is also much easier to practice formula acupuncture than energetic transfer acupuncture if one must treat over one hundred patients in a day—the normal case load of acupuncturists in China. In this sense, TCM acupuncture, like Western medicine, is focused narrowly on syndromes (patterns of disharmony) and does not seek to treat the deeper, human energetic imbalances. Patterns are metaphors or images of imbalance, as Kaptchuk points out in *The Web That Has No Weaver.* One is rarely confronted with an exact pattern, and there is always much more complexity than the mere pattern involved. Many American acupuncturists become aware of this in their own personal struggle with developing a treatment style appropriate and adequate to their American clientele, within three to five years after graduating from school. As Flaws and his colleagues state, this process is to be expected and is full of confusion for the developing practitioners as they work toward a mature practice beyond ideology or mimicry of their teachers.

When the *Essentials* appeared, with the ZangFu syndromes clearly explicated for the first time in English, many American teachers and practitioners began to grow critical of their own earlier training, which usually spoke, more simply it now seemed to them, of Excess, Deficient (and perhaps Cold and Hot) complexes for each organ function. This simpler way of speaking remains in the Japanese traditions, as well as in the Five Element traditional acupuncture approach developed by J. R. Worsley. Flaws et al. criticize Western practitioners of energy transfer acupuncture for shoddy scholarship, which they believe has been at the root of a critique in our own country of acupuncture energetic practices by TCM-style practitioners. Be that as it may, all practitioners trained in this country or Europe or Canada more than ten years ago were far more grounded in energy transfer acupuncture, Five Element strategies, and secondary vessel and Eight Extraordinary Vessel energetics and treatment than those trained in the past five or six years. The *Essentials* and other books emanating from the People's Republic of China have become the major texts for state and national examinations, and all schools are obliged to teach at least the rudiments of TCM as depicted in these dominant texts. In the past ten years the focus has been on translations of the modern Chinese medical texts; yet, as Kaptchuk, who wrote a key TCM text for Americans *(The Web That Has No Weaver)* now states, we must look to other traditions, European and Korean and Vietnamese, which may perhaps have as much or more to offer as we develop a truly Western way of practicing acupuncture suitable to our own patients.[3]

Hence the enormous importance of the works of Matsumoto and Birch, who steadfastly present to Western practitioners and students another way, another view of human energetics and acupuncture, according to ancient *Nan Jing* and modern Japanese traditions.[4]

What is immediately striking about the "asymptomatic" core-energetic approaches presented by Matsumoto and Birch is their focus on somatic, body-energetic zones of the body. Rather than a list of signs and symptoms that include pulse and tongue, this core-energetic approach often places more emphasis on the Hara, the energetic core of the bodymind, with observations about sensitive points or areas and other physical findings. Central to this perspective is a focus on body balance and symmetry, where body signs in one area lead the practitioner to search for associated signs in corresponding somatic energetic zones.

In a seminar at the Tri-State Institute of Traditional Chinese Acupuncture, which I direct, Kiiko Matsumoto discussed the Hara of the Liver deficient condition according to the *Nan Jing*. In addition to signs and symptoms which are related to Liver deficiency in other acupuncture traditions (dislike of wind, headaches, dizziness, myopia, discomfort in the region of the liver, contracted muscles, and difficulty breathing), Matsumoto pointed out the specific point and zone sensitivities of this condition, namely tightness or pain on pressure, or puffiness or resistance in the area directly over and underneath the actual liver organ with similar signs to the left of the navel (Kidney 16–Stomach 25). Also, along with this excess condition in the left colon area, the left Liver meridian shows signs of excess, especially Liver 9 and perhaps Liver 8 and 3, with possible tightness or pain on pressure in the right scapula. It is clear that Matsumoto, and the Japanese practitioners she studied with, are far more open to the energetic body language of their patients than are their TCM peers, who focus solely on pulse, tongue, and a few signs and symptoms in decidedly

Western medical fashion. Some Western practitioners with TCM leanings are critical of this sort of physical focus, decrying what they see as a working-class acupuncture, as opposed to the higher-class TCM approach which is closer to herbology. Such a bias, present in many parts of the Orient as well as the West (in Korea, for example, Doctors of Oriental Medicine take an elitist stance against acupuncturists and feel that only those well versed in herbology practice real medicine, while acupuncturists are seen as mere physical therapists) entirely misses what many American acupuncturists are discovering anew, namely that acupuncture-energetic therapy, and not Oriental pharmacology,[5] is most appropriate for many of the complex functional, psychosomatic, and stress-related disorders of our modern era, bespeaking a split between mind and body along with often severe spiritual distress.

After hearing Kiiko Matsumoto make the above observations regarding Liver deficiency in terms unfamiliar to me (the subtitle of this condition is often Large Intestine excess), adding that in the presence of Large Intestine excess there is often pain or other signs of reactivity on the right side, at the points Large Intestine 4 and 10, I returned to my practice and began to palpate the Hara with greater care, and discovered that many of the patients that I had found to exhibit what is known in TCM as "constrained Liver Qi" did, in fact, show much greater sensitivity at the left Liver 9 and 5 especially, and sometimes at Liver 3; with pain and tightness left of the navel and almost always exquisite sensitivity at right Large Intestine 10, and sometimes 4, along with the familiar tightness at Conception Vessel 10–11 (the locus of constrained Liver energy in the stomach area, predisposing the body to gastric ulcer, stomach distress, or an aneurysm) and under the right ribcage over the Liver area. Needling Liver 8 and 9 on the left (and sometimes Liver 3 or 5 on the left or right, depending on which point was most reactive to palpation) and Large Intestine 4 or 10, if reactive, on the right along with Pericardium 5 or 6 on the left and Conception Vessel 10 or 11, depending again on reactivity, led to a rapid and dramatic amelioration in the stomach tightness and other constrained Liver Qi symptoms.

Every time that Kiiko Matsumoto teaches at our Institute, I find that I, like the other practitioners and students present, am moved to be more aware of body clues in my patients, and also am drawn toward an anecdotal perspective that believes in what is actually experienced as opposed to relying on standard formulas or rigid application of theory.

And therein lies the tremendous importance of Kiiko Matsumoto's own work in this country, as she tries to engage American practitioners in what I see as a phenomenological approach that seeks to be with the person who comes for help, paying close attention to the bodymind as a force field, intervening in terms of the patient's own present condition whether or not it fits some preconceived clinical syndrome or pattern. Working from this perspective (which I learned to do from my early study of Soulie de Morant and Van Nghi almost ten years ago) leads to a great respect for the body as a source of all the information necessary for the practitioner and the patient to work toward bodymind integrity. When a practitioner probes the patient's body carefully, showing that he knows where to palpate, this reinforces the patient's own internal knowledge and awareness that her signs and symptoms are all connected to the same underlying imbalance, and treatment from this bodymind integrative perspective leads the patient to a recollection of being-more-integrated and prods the bodymind—the interacting biosphere of the human body—to restore more appropriate functioning. Such an approach shows great respect for being with the patient in the present, in her actual condition, rather than reducing this phenomenological, living event to a static syndrome or pattern of disharmony. The focus, in such a perspective, is on prodding the bodymind to recognize new *information* and thereby restore normalized *metabolic* functions—to use Manaka's terminology—by intervening in the Real in which the patient finds herself, rather than ignoring the Real for some theoretical perfect pattern. A phenomenological perspective always begins with the body as a living force field whose dynamics must be understood in its own terms. If the patient's body tells us something that is contradictory to the syndromes or patterns we have learned or the theories we have spent hours committing to memory, we must let go of our learning to be truly present at, and open to, the living event before us. As Matsumoto and Birch state so eloquently, "When we palpate a point and find reactiveness, or observe signs and symptoms in an area, it may be a non-standard idea or variant trajectory that provides the clue with which we are able to solve the problem." Their intent here is to emphasize that point locations or meridian trajectories are never exactly as portrayed in texts, which present a kind of common denominator of location, and that the careful practitioner, working from the phenomenological perspective,[6] will carefully palpate and observe the patient, going with what he finds rather than force the findings into neatly demarcated, learned theories. Thus, a practitioner committed to continuous learning will be open to other theories and discussion of human energetics but, ultimately, will leave theories behind if the patient's actual state of affairs demands a different understanding. It is this openness to the actual state of the patient's health that has led the Japanese practitioners studied by Matsumoto and Birch to observe tenderness at left Liver 9 in Liver deficient conditions, a fact easily confirmed by any practitioner who elects to carefully palpate his patients' bodies.

In Manaka's approach, which has greatly influenced

Matsumoto's own treatment style, "both sender and receiver are essential."[7] The practitioner who works to be attuned to the event before him and the patient in his actual living energetic state form an intimate unit in the phenomenological bodymind energetic approach, leaving no room for an elitist stance, still present in some Oriental medical herbal approaches, where the doctor coldly palpates the radial artery, looks at the tongue, and asks a few questions, then makes a diagnostic pronouncement and writes orders to be followed by the compliant patient.

In their newest work, *Hara: Reflections on the Sea*, Matsumoto and Birch provide the information necessary for grounding *acupuncture palpation* on a perspective of the body energetic that focuses on fascial constrictions and interferences in connective tissue. Such constrictions, referred to as "Kori," which we shall return to in Chapter 8, can be released by acupuncture in such a way as to free up lymph and venous circulation as well as the arterial and nervous systems, thereby restoring organ functions as well.

It may well be that American acupuncturists, influenced by traditions other than TCM, such as those studied and presented by Matsumoto and Birch in their invaluable books, will bring the Self[8] back to the practice of acupuncture—both the Self of the practitioner as it works to listen and observe and be present in ways not common to everyday being-in-the-world, and the Self of the patient as it strives to be more integrated and whole. In this way, acupuncture-energetic therapy will become more than a practice to treat illness according to standardized prescriptions, as in the American TCM approaches. It will expand to realize, as Matsumoto and Birch emphasize, "that events in a living human will often confound theory."[9]

5

Organ-Functional Energetics

A BEHAVIORAL PERSPECTIVE ON ZANGFU

The influence of TCM (ZangFu) acupuncture on my teaching and practice, as on that of most American educators and practitioners over the past several years, has been great. The TCM diagnostic process, by means of the Eight Principles and simplified tongue and pulse confirmations, coupled with a more detailed and precise picture of ZangFu (organ-functional) energetic disturbances, made it much easier to teach beginners the basics of Chinese medical diagnosis.

I have found it necessary in teaching my students at the Tri-State Institute of Traditional Chinese Acupuncture to integrate the Eight Principles into a more carefully spelled out process of diagnosis and treatment planning that does not forget the Five Phases and the role of meridian disturbances. These factors must be taken into account in any treatment plan, but are left out of TCM acupuncture teachings that have reached the West, where the only significant meridian disorder is cold in the Liver meridian![1]

Where the earlier French teachings had lead one to look for excess, deficient, hot, and cold patterns for each Zang and Fu, the TCM portrayal of what Kaptchuk terms Patterns of Disharmony made it clear that not every organ-function had the same sorts of disorders. Hence, rising Fire disorders do not occur everywhere, but rather in Liver, Gallbladder, Heart, and Stomach functions. Likewise, deficient Yang patterns were frequent in the Kidney, Spleen, and Heart functions, and far more rare in the other functions. This specificity helps one understand more accurately the actual incidence of disturbance in the various organ-functions, and also makes it possible to translate Western diseases into organ-functional patterns in a much more useful way than with Five Element theory or the older hot/cold—empty/full way of speaking of the organ-functions.

The weakness of the TCM acupuncture perspective, as I see it, is in overly medicalizing the practice of acupuncture. This happens every time a student or practitioner thinks, for example, that in treating someone with hypertension who displays a deficiency of Yin of the Kidneys, he is treating the hypertension and not the Yin of the Kidneys. In this case, he will be narrowing his attention to the blood pressure, rather than focusing on the Yin of the Kidneys.

The other problem with the TCM, ZangFu approach is that it often leads one to forget that meridian disturbances can occur *without* ZangFu disturbances. Like practitioners trained by Worsley, who treat primarily the regular meridian system and the "Officials" (ZangFu seen in a more psychological way than in TCM), TCM practitioners almost always treat the ZangFu and primarily utilize the regular meridians as their site for the selection of local and distal points. There is nothing inherently wrong with this basic focus on the regular meridians and ZangFu, but I find it necessary, from the combined influence of the French and Japanese teachings mentioned above, to pay constant attention to the secondary vessels that constitute the energetics of the surface, while at the same time seeking to return the bodymind to the integrity of the primal energetics of the extraordinary vessel system, in order to successfully treat my clients. The Eight Extraordinary Vessels are *pre–organ-functional* (Pre-ZangFu; pre-Officials); the secondary vessels are more superficial than the organ-functions, and serve to protect these functions. To treat without paying attention to *what came before* the organ-functions, rendering them possible (the Eight Extraordinary Vessels as the precondition for the organ-functions) and to *what protects* these functions (the secondary vessels as armor) reveals a bias toward the organ-functions at the expense of the meridian system that supports them. After all, as the French teachings point out, the ZangFu are merely more concentrated zones of energetic activity of the meridian system itself.

In addition to integrating the TCM Eight Principle diagnosis within a larger, problem-solving process of treatment planning that does not ignore the Five Phases and meridian energetics, I have found it necessary and beneficial to reformulate these patterns of ZangFu disharmony as *reaction patterns* in line with modern behavioral stress research and practice. In this reformulation, a person does not *have* constrained Liver Qi as he might have hyperthyroidism, as a disease or disorder of a rather objective sort (that one can "catch" or "get" and "get rid of" or "control"). Rather (and I believe this is more in line with the ancient Chinese concept of the interaction between Man, Heaven, and Earth), a person behaves in the world in such a way, owing to predisposition to dysfunction in certain imbalanced energetic functions or zones (primarily Liver or Spleen in the above example) and *in response* to environmental stressors and internal emotional states or events, that he develops constriction, in this case in the diaphragm and pit of the stomach, leading to a complex series of reactions depending on the type of stressor, the specific situation, and his own predispositions. To educate the client about his *way of behaving in a constrained Liver Qi fashion* is very different from thinking to oneself, and perhaps even telling him, that *he has constrained Liver Qi*. While the latter way of presenting TCM patterns to the patient is decidedly medical and medicalizing (energetic states and reactions are not seen as such, but as syndromes more like Western syndromes), the former, behavioral perspective establishes a client-centered therapeutic approach in which the goal of bodymind integration is coupled with a focus on improving one's ability to react to stressors, cope with the events of life, and remain more energetically centered throughout, placing responsibility for change with the client.

In order to make it easier to reformulate the TCM patterns of disharmony as *energetic reaction patterns*, I returned to an earlier interest in classic psychosomatics (Groddeck, Deutsch, Dunbar, Alexander, and others). To my delight, these Western psychoanalysts, who were interested in bodymind dynamics, often perceived patterns such as "diaphragmatic neuroses" (which correlates with what TCM acupuncture terms "constrained Liver Qi") that were akin to the patterns of disharmony of the Chinese view. In their conception of *vegetative* or *organ neuroses*, they had developed essentially the same notion as the early Chinese of organ-functional dynamics, that constituted the basis for a dynamic, functional medicine. All that was missing in their system was an understanding of the somatic energetics that accompanied the psychodynamics they had so carefully charted. While they hoped endocrinology or other new branches of medicine would finally explain the somatic dynamics of these functional "neuroses," they would have done better to research the Chinese functional energetic concepts. In Chapters 4–10 of *Bodymind Energetics* I move from a summary of this classic psychosomatic view to a bodymind-energetic approach to acupuncture that juxtaposes Chinese organ-functional and energetic perspectives with

Western psychosomatic understandings. This reformulation of organ-functional patterns makes it easier to understand and explain my own *imaging* process with my clients. As I develop a contract with them in the first session, to the effect that their disturbance or uneasiness or illness will be imaged in bodymind energetic terms—with the intention of mending the body/mind splits underlying this disturbance—by prodding the body energetic to remember how to function more appropriately by stimulating specific energetic pathways and zones, I can easily make the nature of this imaging clear if I bring in the psychosomatic, vegetative perspective, thereby grounding the ZangFu understanding in terms more familiar to Westerners. An example of this sort of imaging concerning common stress reaction patterns I observe daily in my stressed New York clients, and also in those suffering from immune deficiency disorders, appears in Chapter 6.

In brief, the simplicity and accuracy of the TCM approach to organ-functional diagnosis as well as its understanding of the major patterns of the ZangFu (derived from the observations of countless treatments over thousands of years and therefore representing a highly reliable picture against which to begin to measure our clients' complaints), when reformulated in behavioral terms (reaction patterns vs. patterns of disharmony), is an essential aspect of my approach to acupuncture therapy.[2]

6

Diaphragmatic Reactivity and Stress Reactions: An Acupuncture-Energetic View of Immune Dysfunction

A recurrent sign I have encountered in a large number of clients with Chronic Fatigue Syndrome*, AIDS, and ARC (AIDS-related complex), is extreme reactivity in the diaphragm during palpation. At times clients are well aware of these zones as an area where they hold stress; at other times not. In either case even the most gentle palpation of the region underneath the ribs in the front, and the corresponding zone in the back, elicits spasm of the muscles that sometimes wraps around the entire zone. Given the importance of the diaphragmatic and abdominal zones in acupuncture energetics, this finding helps point a way toward imaging these immune deficiency disorders in energetic terms, thereby facilitating their understanding and treatment with acupuncture therapy.

Figure 1 shows diagrams illustrating the diaphragmatic zones in question, with certain reflex zones that appear to be intimately connected, in certain instances, with this diaphragmatic constriction.

* Also known as Chronic Fatigue and Immune Dysfunction Syndrome (CFIDS) and, formerly, as Chronic Epstein-Bar Virus (CEBV).

FIGURE 1

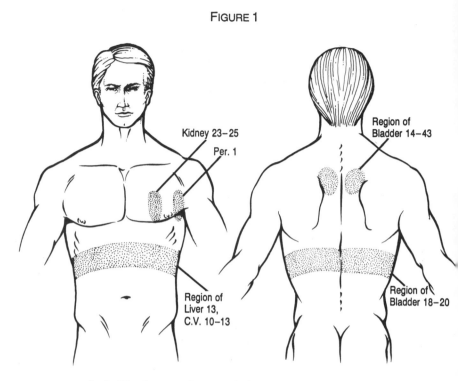

Kidney 23-25
Per. 1
Region of Liver 13, C.V. 10-13
Region of Bladder 14-43
Region of Bladder 18-20

Left: *Diaphragmatic constriction—abdominal zone.*
Right: *Diaphragmatic constriction—back zone.*

In attempting to understand immune deficiency disorders in acupuncture energetic terms, we must begin by exploring the role of Wei (defensive) energy, which nourishes the skin surface and strengthens "the fabric of the skin as a result of the appropriate opening and closing of the pores."[1] Wei energy thus creates the defensive barrier against external pathogenic factors and environmental stress, playing the role of psychosomatic "character armor" as well.[2] It protects deep internal organ-energetic functions by preventing the invasion of external pathogenic stressors.

What is often forgotten in acupuncture discussion is that at the deep level "Wei energy plays a role in the functioning of the diaphragm, at the level of the mesenteric formations of the thorax and the belly,"[3] as the late Dr. Jean Schatz stresses, and thereby connects with the organs. Wei energy unites the peritoneum, the pleura, and the pericardium, and thus has a connection "with the pre-eminent role that Western medicine presently grants to the connective tissues . . . constituted to work principally on the defense of the thoraco-abdominal viscera."[4]

In traditional acupuncture-energetic physiology, the Liver energetic function is responsible for the free flow of energy through the organism, on both a physical and mental plane. If Liver energy is flowing properly, the musculature, the region of the ribs (ruled by the Liver energetic function), and the behavior and moods of the individual will be harmonious and even. The spirit of the Liver has to do with the "giving of images," the "function of imaging," and the "plans and outlines brought to the individual in his hereditary endowment," known collectively as Hun.[5] As Schatz and his colleagues conclude, the Hun of the Liver function supplies the hereditary code whereby humans have the power to call upon images of functioning at all levels of the organism. That the Liver meridian also supplies the energy for the eyes and sight further underscores the primal role of the Liver in body imaging.[6]

If we perceive of acupuncture therapy not as direct, objective treatment of disease and dysfunction but rather as a *prod to the bodymind to remember how to restore appropriate functioning* to heal itself, then it is clear that this prodding has something fundamental to do with activating the Liver to call up the appropriate functional images in the case of vegetative disturbance. To take this behavioral perspective a step further, in line with modern stress theories, acupuncture serves as a minor stressor to activate the sympathetic nervous system. In doing so, it activates not only the adrenals (the mother of the Liver in acupuncture energetic physiology) and Liver, but the entire function of imaging. Given that the Liver and Pericardium (or Heart Protector) are both the same great meridian (Jueyin), it is clear that stimulation of the Liver also stimulates the Pericardium function. The latter rules the region between the breasts, namely C.V. 17, and, according to Dr. Lavier, "plays an essential role in the physiology of the sympathetic nervous system."[7]

Under chronic stress, the adrenals (Yang of the Kidneys), Liver, and musculature of the chest and upper back (Pericardium energetic zone) become permanently constricted. This often leads to patterns similar to the Organ functional pattern known in Traditional Chinese Medicine as "constrained Liver Qi." There may be agitated emotional states, inappropriate anger, constriction in the pit of the stomach and diaphragm, chest constriction, and even throat constriction ("plum-pit feeling"). This constriction, over time, may lead to a localized lesion in the pit of the stomach (C.V. 10–13), namely an ulcer; rising "Fire" disorders as can be found in hiatus hernia (functional or organic, with the incidence of functional disorders of the diaphragm on the increase if my experience is any indication), reflux esophagitis, and esophageal constriction. Or, shifting into parasympathetic reaction patterns, there may be patterns of "Liver invading the Spleen-Pancreas" leading to disturbance in the latter. From an acupuncture-energetic perspective, this set of stress reaction patterns calls into play the entire Middle Heater, the energetics of Jueyin (Liver and Pericardium) and the major (and possibly first embryologically, according to Schatz) extraordinary vessel Chung Mo, which rises up through the regions energized by the Liver and Kidney Yang, connecting peritoneum, pleura, and pericardium, and serving as the foundation upon which all organ

FIGURE 2

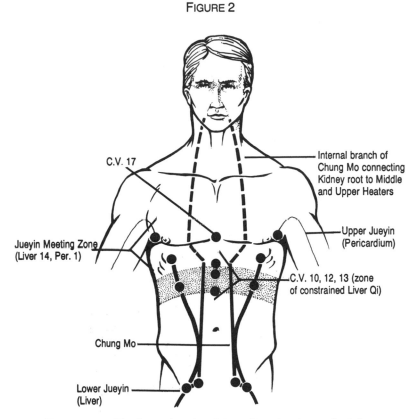

Treatment: *To these local points, when tender, select from Jueyin, Chung Mo, and Yinweimo points: Spleen 4, Per. 6, Liver 3, 5, 8, 9, depending on reactivity.*

functions develop. Figure 2 illustrates this complex energetic web of reactions.

Now, the diaphragmatic (constrained Liver Qi) patterns evoked above are extremely common, along with panic disorder variants connecting weakness in the Kidney energy (at C.V. 6–7) with Pericardium constriction and Chung Mo obstruction, which might best be visualized as adrenal exhaus-

FIGURE 3

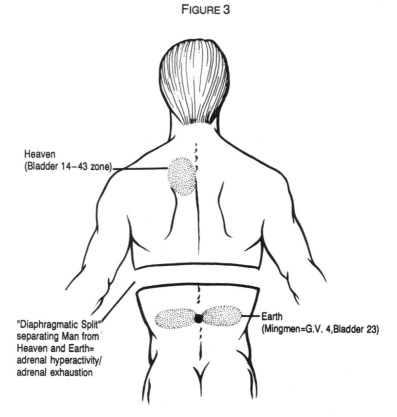

Heaven
(Bladder 14–43 zone)

"Diaphragmatic Split"
separating Man from
Heaven and Earth=
adrenal hyperactivity/
adrenal exhaustion

Earth
(Mingmen=G.V. 4,Bladder 23)

Treatment: To these local areas, where tender, add Kid. 2 and 3; Per. 4, 5, 6

tion patterns whereby Kidney Yang loses its harmonious relationship with Ming Men (the original spark of life) and the Heart, mediated by the Pericardium.[8] Given that the third (foot or cubit) position of the pulses on the right is palpated by acupuncturists both to ascertain the functioning of the Heart Protector (Pericardium) in the Upper Heater, and the Yang of the Kidneys in the Lower Heater, a mediating role uniting in a complex fashion Pericardium and Kidney Yang, and Upper and Lower Heaters, must be conceptualized.[9] I believe that the

FIGURE 4

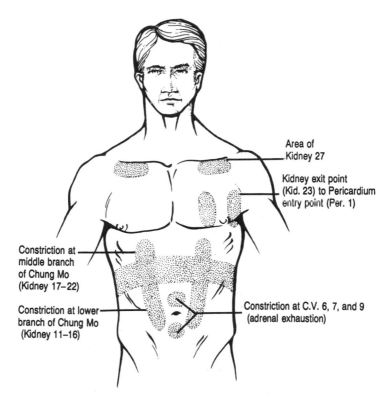

Area of
Kidney 27

Kidney exit point
(Kid. 23) to Pericardium
entry point (Per. 1)

Constriction at
middle branch
of Chung Mo
(Kidney 17–22)

Constriction at lower
branch of Chung Mo
(Kidney 11–16)

Constriction at C.V. 6, 7, and 9
(adrenal exhaustion)

Treatment: *To these local areas, where tender, add Spleen 4
(right); Per. 6 (left); Kidney 2, 3, or 9 = Yinweimo/Chung Mo*

myriad panic syndromes emerging in modern stressful envi-
ronments can be understood energetically as a result of
diaphragmatic constriction straining the middle branch of
Chung Mo, leading to disruption and even a relative break
between upper and lower regions of the body (Kidney Yang
and Pericardium). These syndromes serve as the precondition
for the development of lowered immunity and chronic fatigue
syndrome. Figures 3 and 4 show suggested treatment patterns.

FIGURE 5

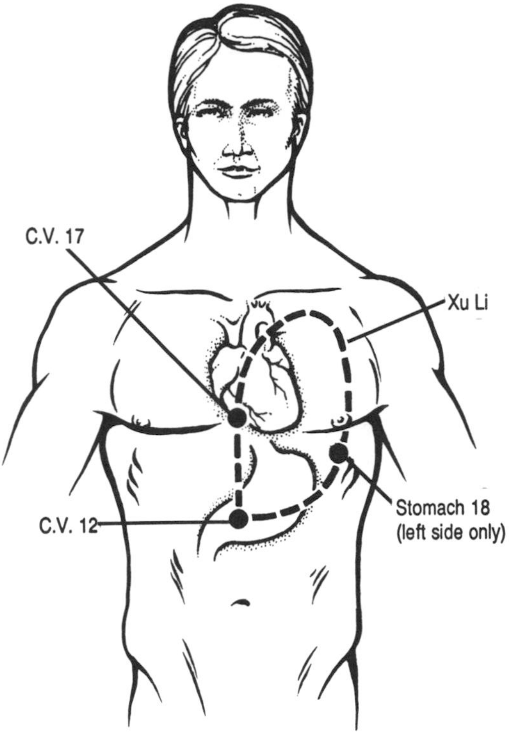

C.V. 17

Xu Li

C.V. 12

Stomach 18
(left side only)

Treatment: *Disperse St. 18, left; free up C.V. 12, 17; St. 13, 14–16; and, if red above the throat, St. 4 and St. 8, bilaterally.*

In some cases this disruption in Chung Mo leads to Stomach Fire Blazing taking the path of Xu Li, the Luo of the Stomach that leads Stomach Fire into the Heart and Pericardium zones, with redness and stagnation from the level of the nipples to St. 12–13; or to St. 9; or even St. 8. See figure 5.

Returning to our point of departure regarding immune deficiency disorders, far less common are the patterns— similar in most details to those above—in which spastic diaphragmatic reactivity is also present, as outlined at the beginning of this essay. Informed by the above discussion, might it be that those suffering from AIDS, ARC, CFS, and CEBV (as well as other immune deficiency disorders yet to be isolated and named) are those whose entire Wei defensive energy system, comprising character armor, adrenals (Kidney Yang), Liver, and Pericardium functions and Chung Mo activity (feeding all vegetative functions as well as serving as their precondition), is severely depleted?

Preliminary work with these clients seems to point in this direction. Acupuncture therapists working with AIDS and ARC clients report the need to focus on the Yin and Yang Root of the Kidneys and the Middle Heater constantly, and the oft-cited use of Bladder 43 (Gaohuang) shows the importance of treating the Pericardium and the "region between the breasts" (thought to activate the production of bone marrow and prod the entire immunological system). This is also true in the treatment of Chronic Fatigue Syndrome.

If the diaphragm is as important in the functioning of the immune (Wei–defensive) system as acupuncture energetics seems to illustrate, the sign of extreme reactivity in the pit of the abdomen and diaphragm in patients suffering from immune deficiency disorders is of great significance and may point those working with such clients toward stress reduction therapies that free up the diaphragm. Many self-help–oriented clients with these disorders have found that diaphragmatic breathing, stress reduction techniques to free up the musculature (the muscular meridian level ruled by Wei defensive energy constituting the character armor as well), proper diet to nourish the organism (and allow the Middle Heater to work properly, rather than being overworked), and visualization (especially of proper spleen immunological functioning) are key factors in their own maintenance of control over the progress of their disorders and a state of increased well-being.

In the Orient, and especially in Japan, the importance of the diaphragm and the area under its control (the Hara) has not been forgotten. In the West, where constricted, shallow breathing and a pulled-in Middle Heater and diaphragm is the norm, it is not surprising that disorders develop out of this diaphragmatic constriction. Perhaps this explains the amazing effects of simple meditation techniques discovered by Westerners only recently—discovered, perhaps, out of an intuitive sense of the need to open up the diaphragm and breathe in an unconstricted manner. If this is true, the benefit of Qi Gong (now gaining recognition in the West as it regains respect in China) will be of extreme importance.[10]

Acupuncture therapists, practitioners of Oriental medicine, and body workers might do well to pay more attention to this diaphragmatic zone, therefore educating their clients about the energetics of this crucial, middle zone of the bodymind. In prodding the bodymind: to remember the primal functions of Chung Mo (and the potential for all other vegetative functions); to strengthen the Liver energetic function and the Jueyin Great meridian unit (Liver-Pericardium) while freeing up the diaphragm; and to restore the normal relationship between the adrenals and the Pericardium; acupuncture therapists are capable of guiding the individual toward parasympathetic relaxation that enables the bodymind to set right the imaging of functions. In this way, and of course only if the individual recognizes the effects of stress on his body's reaction patterns and well-being and takes responsibility for moderating his life to avoid overly stressful situations, the individual might be able to connect with the primal potential for healthy functioning and catalyze his will to be well in the myriad stress conditions that threaten the functioning of the immune system.

PART III

Acupuncture Treatment Staging

7

Acupuncture Imaging: Where to Begin, How to Proceed

Many acupuncture educators, myself included, have failed to some extent to clearly lay out the actual treatment planning process we use. While we may teach treatment planning in the context of Eight Principles or Five Elements, we often forget to clarify that in real clinical practice, no one proceeds as the books say. Instead, each practitioner adopts what might be called an idiosyncratic style. While recent graduates of acupuncture schools may follow their teachings rather closely, they will eventually develop a personal way of selecting: a place to begin, establishing priorities in the treatment planning, determining followups if changes occur that were not foreseen, and so on. If their own studies do not prepare students for this eventuality, they may develop a personal style without being aware of what the style consists of. They may come to value certain patterns of treatment over others, for example, focusing more on the relationship between Qi and Blood than on the Five Elements or the levels of energetics of the bodymind, unaware that in choosing where to begin and how to proceed, they are leaving out other ways of perceiving the clinical data and ordering a treatment.

As stated in Chapter 2, acupuncture therapists in the West perform an *imaging* when they meet with their clients, especially in the initial interview, because they are taking the details from the client's report and reconceptualizing it—whether they share this reconceptualization with their clients or not—as an *energetic phenomenon* requiring an energetic treatment. If the practitioner is unclear about the nature of his imaging process (and his own priorities, biases, even prejudices regarding this process) he will not be able to be clear with his client. His choice of words and mode of expression may then undermine the intent of the acupuncture treatment itself. Ideally, imaging empowers a person to perceive his problem in a new light and from a different vantage point, serving as a catalyst to change. When we acupuncture therapists perform an *acupuncture imaging*, I do not see how we can maximize the effects of acupuncture unless we are clear with ourselves and our clients that we are reformulating their complaints into the language and perspectives of acupuncture energetics and Oriental medicine (in terms of a view of the body as traversed by energy gradients and zones of concentration, a relationship between the body's elemental material—Qi, Blood, Body Fluids, Shen—and organ-functional relationships).

In a very real sense, then, I know that I am asking each new client: "Are you willing to look at this problem of yours, which your medical doctor has diagnosed in medical or psychological terms, in the functional, *dynamic*, and *energetic* terms of traditional acupuncture and Oriental medicine, where body and mind are subsumed under the broader category of bodymind energetics? In place of the 'either it is physical or it is psychological,' are you willing to view it as energetic, dynamic, functional, where physical, mental, and even spiritual signs and symptoms can occur together at the same time?"

I take this *imaging* a step further by educating the person about what I perceive in the acupuncture-energetic terms that I use. Rather than make an acupuncture or Oriental medical *diagnosis* (attributing a pathological condition to an Element, meridian, or organ-energetic function), I offer a phenomenological *description* of the person's energetics as I see it, while palpating the points and zones to elicit confirming responses (a bodily felt sense) from the client.

Example: Your doctor has diagnosed your problem as nervous stomach and functional hiatus hernia and has sent you to me because I specialize in psychosomatic disorders. Your chiropractor also treats you for a sacral misalignment and TMJ syndrome. Now, when your doctor says "psychosomatic" he doubtless means "psychologically caused", or "non-organic," whereas when I use the term I mean that many disorders have psychological and physical components which must be addressed at the same time. I treat disorders as a mind/body split, an event that has disrupted the bodymind's capacity for integration and harmony. In your case, you appear to hold an enormous amount of tension and stress in your trapezius, jaws, temples, diaphragm, and outer aspect of the legs. What appear to be different problems (sacral misalignment, stomach distress, a constriction in the pit of the stomach that sometimes goes up to the throat, and tightness and clicking in the jaws spreading to the temples) are really manifestations of one energetic zone, in this case the Lesser Yang zone of the Gallbladder and Triple Heater meridians, with problems arising at the points where the energies of this zone are most concentrated (this said, after the intake and while palpating the client on the table, *with accentuated pressure*, on palpation of the Gallbladder and Triple Heater pathways, of T.H. 5, T.H. 15, G.B. 21, T.H. 16, Anmian, G.B. 20, G.B. 13–14, G.B. 3–T.H. 22, T.H. 23 to G.B. 1, and then to G.B. 24, Liver 13 and 14, C.V. 10,–12, G.B. 26,–29, 31, 34, 38,–41).

Palpating the affected zone while providing an energetic description of the zone *leads* the client into a bodymind energetic *image*. *Pacing* my comments and my palpation so that intellectual understanding and bodily awareness coincide with bodily felt reactions of the client to the description and palpation helps me to lead the client into the bodymind energetic imaging of his complaint in a way that empowers the client and maintains control in his hands, because all significant information emanates from his bodily felt awareness. Such awareness, which we all carry deep inside, is a preverbal, organic and visceral, largely unconscious, right-brain way of processing the world. While the client might retort that this sort of pressure would hurt anyone at those points, that the pain at the top of his foot is insignificant, and what, anyway, does it have to do with his major problem, he knows, at some deeper, older, earlier (even prenatal in some instances) level, that these zones where he is reactive are all part of a whole, connected, *patterned response* that forms a single unit. He often has had vague recollections of this patterned response, knowing it was connected all along. These kinds of bodily felt recollections and recognitions are commonplace in the practice of any acupuncturist or Oriental medical bodyworker (shiatsuist, acupressurist) who is in the habit of palpating points and meridian zones *during the evaluation* (as opposed to merely palpating to locate the point for needling) with clients exclaiming, "How did you know about that point that is always killing me?" or "When you press that point, I want to cry and yell at the same time!" or "What is that point; it creates a knife-like pain all the way up to my stomach!" or "That place always hurts me when I get my headaches" or "I get a fleeting feeling of nausea in that area before I have one of my dizzy spells"—and so on.

Proceeding further with this client, I point out that the muscular rigidity and reactivity along the Lesser Yang zone seem to be serving as a shield, an armor to protect a deeper deficiency, in the Yin pair to this zone, namely the Absolute Yin, Liver (and Pericardium to a lesser extent) energetic zone.

Palpating these deficient pathways, I pace my comments to a more gentle, supportive palpation and reactions from the client, to lead the client more deeply into the bodymind-energetic realm we have both agreed to explore, where I am like a guide who knows the territory and the characteristics of its manifold terrains, and he is the explorer in search of lost connections, seeking bodymind integrity.

When I palpate the Yang, muscular reactive zones (character armor, as it were), I emphasize, by the nature of my deep pressure, the severity of the muscular tightness until the client acknowledges this muscular defensiveness (I make comments like "You sure don't hold any *tension there*, do you?" or "It looks like nothing could get through *that!"*). The use of humorous, paradoxical language and tones is appropriate when these muscular zones are palpated since the client is well protected here and can stand some prodding. If the timing seems right, I take the opportunity of this palpation to perform deep acupressure to release some of the muscular rigidity, both to ready the area for insertion of needles (needling directly into severe muscle spasms and trigger points can create very negative reactions) and to provide some immediate relief, to see what happens at the deeper weak zone once energy from the surface is freed up.

In palpating the Yin, deficient zones (Absolute Yin, Liver in this case), I use a more supportive pressure and combine this with nurturing, supportive comments ("This is a bit cold, isn't it? Let's see what happens when I place my hands here to warm it up" or "This feels a bit empty, doesn't it? Let's try to prod the Liver meridian to move energy here."), emphasizing constricted areas, full of excessive energy, as they compensate for the weak areas (focusing on how we can pull from the excess area rather than focusing on the emptiness) and warm zones that coincide with cold ones (enjoining the client to imagine for a moment the warmth from the warm areas moving to the cold area). Whereas the palpation of the Yang muscular zones-of-holding focuses on the exact pathways and points of concentration of energy, palpation of the Yin zones (the front of the body, and the inner aspects of the arms and legs) focuses on the Hara—the bodymind's energetic core—which is much more vulnerable than the Yang zone. I also palpate key distal points along the Yin zones to assess meridian energetic blockages and to confirm my working hypothesis of the disorder (Liver 3, 5, 8, 9, 13, 14, Bladder 18, C.V. 10–11, and Pericardium 5–6 in this case).

In the above case I would point out how much more disturbed it feels under the right ribcage, over the Liver, and at Bl. 17, 18, 19 on the right side in the back. Also I would point out reactivities in associated areas while sharing with the client my view of the stress response from an acupuncture perspective, where the weakness, leading to constriction, in the Liver function encroaches upon the Spleen, weakens the Middle Heater, and leads to energetic accumulation and "rebellious movement" up the Chung Mo (the reflex associated with hiatus hernia in this case). I would ask whether the client ever drank a lot or abused drugs or had hepatitis, making it clear that while sensitivity in this area does not necessarily imply disorder of the actual Liver organ, it could. I would make suggestions about how to change the diet, and suggest some self-help techniques to relax the diaphragm (the "constrained Liver Qi"). I would also mention that in classical psychosomatic theory, this would be called a "diaphragmatic neurosis," explaining that this *readiness of the diaphragm to react* is what sets the stage for the nervous stomach and hiatus hernia. I make it clear that the acupuncture will not be treating the actual medical disorders diagnosed by the doctor, but rather this "readiness to react," by prodding the Lesser Yang and Absolute Yin pathways to support the Liver function to remember how to act more appropriately. "The needles, then, are not treating your complaints," I will add, "but are prodding your body and mind to remember how to circulate and flow in these zones, thereby releasing obstructions, warming up cold areas, and freeing up constricted ones, to allow for better circulation of the body's nutrients to this overused or neglected zone." I make my initial selection as to whether to focus on the constricted Lesser Yang zones or support the weak Liver energetic function based on the client's wishes ("Would you like to start with these tight areas in your neck and jaw and stomach, or begin by supporting the weak area directly, moving on to these zones later if they do not free up once this area is strengthened?"). This gives the client the *freedom* to choose (and they always do make a choice when offered the chance) in a way that keeps him in *control* of the change that will occur (some people want to keep their muscular tensions but cannot bear their weak areas and the symptoms and complaints that arise from them, whereas others need and want immediate relief from this tension, which itself will already lead to strengthening of the weak areas which would grow weaker or become traumatized if treated directly). In either case, I will always utilize a few points in the other zone, to remind the body of the interaction between the Yang reactions (coping mechanisms) and the Yin predispositions to dysfunction (constitution). (In this case, if I treated points along Lesser Yang to free up the jaw, neck, and diaphragm, I would also use a few points to support Absolute Yin, like Per. 6 and Liver 5, for example, and vice versa.) Once the needles are in, I would direct this client to close his eyes and relax (said with slowed-down, relaxed breathing on my part) and feel and sense his breathing moving through the affected zones where the needles have been placed, with the breathing moving into the tightness in the pit of the stomach (the constrained Liver zone) to open the diaphragm and restore a free-flowing energy throughout the body. These comments, of course, are based upon the normal functioning of the Liver function and Official, and are made to consolidate the effect of the needles. As the client's awareness is on this energetic zone of the diaphragm (imaged in energetic terms), his deeper intention to heal this area, mend the body/mind split, and achieve bodymind integrity is catalyzed. As a catalyst, the acupuncture imaging process gives the client the freedom to change. The result of the treatment might, as is sometimes the case, temporarily lead to further constriction in this zone, or even greater disturbance in the Liver and Lesser Yang zones than before, in which case the acupuncture therapist has to determine carefully whether the treatment was at fault or whether this is resistance emanating from the client's will to remain ill.[1] It is entirely possible to give what appears to be a "correct" treatment, but undo it with one's comments to the patient. My favorite example is when a practitioner, in response to the client's question about what will happen during the treatment says, "Nothing, just relax."

When the needles are out and the client is ready to leave, I explain that I want him to pay attention, without worrying about it, to *any* changes that arise—whether physical or emotional, improvements or aggravations—explaining that any of the areas and functions associated with Lesser Yang and Absolute Yin zones could go through changes, and that this will enable us to hone in more precisely on the next treatment. This open-ended comment maintains the imaging in the bodymind-energetic realm and catalyzes the client's capacities for change *by making no diagnosis or prediction*.

In this decidedly phenomenological fashion, I attempt to educate every new client to a bodymind-energetic understanding and somatic awareness of his complaint. This education or guidance is behavioral and is aimed at empowering him to relearn/remember/recollect proper bodymind-energetic functioning. My bias is that we all were given to understand this from birth (probably even intrauterinally, as some modern investigators are postulating) and that awareness at this level is necessary for fundamental and lasting change to occur. As practitioners are coming to recognize more and more, it is essential to prod not only, or not especially, the intellectual memory—which many forms of psychotherapy focus on to the exclusion of somatic awareness—but also the *body's recollection of being*.[2]

As the client leaves we are both clear about the *context* for our work together, and he leaves with a fresh perspective of his complaints that postulates a unity of mind and body conceived of as a dynamic, energetic, interactive realm full of potential for change. This is a dynamic, functional context that empowers a person by providing him with an *energetic story* —a primal energetic myth, as it were—that holds out great promise for transformation, growth, and healing, provided the client wants it and is willing to participate actively rather than be passively treated. A knowledge of one's bodymind energetics, I believe, enables a person to have *control* of the Self and is in the service of the *freedom* to *change*. Control, freedom, and change are the three key terms of health psychology and modern psychosomatics, and together define what health really is. As an ancient body therapy, acupuncture energetics and the palpation process as defined above are a powerful prod to awaken this somatic awareness, this bodily felt recollection of being that would appear to be at the core of any profound changes, if one agrees, as I do, with Eugene Gendlin, a psychologist and phenomenologist who revealed the crucial role of this bodily felt sense in psychological transformation in psychotherapy.[3]

8

Bodymind-Energetic
Palpation

SOMATIC ENERGETIC AWARENESS AS A GROUNDING FORCE

Many American acupuncture therapists do not palpate the body in any significant way. A quick check of a few Mu and Shu points on the initial visit is often the extent of the palpation, thus delaying the possibility for a somatic energetic awareness on the patient's part until the needles are inserted. What this does, often against the therapist's intent, is to shift the locus of control away from the client to the practitioner. Since the client has no chance of reacting to the evaluation process somatically, no chance of sensing and feeling what the acupuncture therapist is explaining, the context of the treatment can rarely be other than the orthodox doctor–patient relationship, in which the doctor knows what is wrong and how to fix it and the client is a passive recipient of treatment. While some practitioners do not relate to their clients at all, and still treat effectively (granted, insertion of needles provokes great changes, even with neophytes) we are speaking here not just of alleviation of symptoms, but of an education process in which the client learns how to regain and maintain health, preferably using acupuncture only by choice rather than depending on it.

Palpation as described in Chapter 7 brings the client, and his bodymind awareness, into the center of the process, starting the healing process with the interview rather than with the insertion of needles. What is said by any health practitioner during the intake can prod the *placebo capacity*, as some are now coming to term it (the capacity for self-healing with minimal outside intervention), *or can hinder it severely!* While Asian practitioners do not teach about or make use of the placebo capacity and bodymind awareness in most instances, we in the West must, it seems to me, if we are to place acupuncture in the forefront of new models of health rather than relegate it to a possibly outdated pathological, medical/ medicalizing model. It takes time to palpate in the way I describe, but this time is all part of the healing process and part of the treatment, and sets the stage for a powerful change once the needles are inserted. This palpation/evaluation/imaging process often provokes changes in and of itself, with no needling. It also cuts down tremendously on the number of treatments a person needs. Except for trauma or acute pain, which may require several treatments in close succession, I tend to treat someone two or three times at first, with a week between each session. Then, after the second or third treatment, I give the next treatment two or sometimes even three weeks later, another treatment a month later, a seasonal followup session a few months later, and three or four treatments a year if the client is using acupuncture for health maintenance as well as for a specific set of complaints. This is easily only one half the number of treatments I used to perform, with better results overall than when I treated more frequently. I believe this is because I have learned how to capitalize on the treatment process by placing the client's capacities, not my treatment, at the center. I believe that once prodded, the bodymind can go on to heal itself with very little outside interference. So I interfere and intervene as little as possible. I have found that the most significant changes often occur after a break of two or three weeks *when the client is not being treated.* If we acupuncture therapists treat too much and too often, I believe we make our clients dependent upon the treatments and impede their own capacity for self-healing and bodymind integration.

Palpation is also a way of bringing closeness into the therapeutic process and lets the client know that what you know is *real* (touching him at Liver 3 and C.V. 10–11 and saying 'You sure hold it all in there, don't you?' is far more convincing and powerful, and immediately therapeutic, than diagnostically pronouncing, "You have constrained Liver Qi"). The Real of somatic energetic awareness touches deep layers of knowing and opens the way for the needles to be catalysts, rather than invasions, in the territory of the client's bodymind energetics.

An image came to me as I was trying to explain to my students that Matsumoto was working from a very different place than do TCM acupuncturists. While the latter focus on organ patterns (ZangFu), Matsumoto is concerned instead with the body constrictions that lie behind these organ dysfunctions.

The image was this. Imagine you have been called in by the traffic authority in New York City to solve the traffic problem. You forget to ask what the nature of this traffic problem is, but assume that there must be a terrible accumulation of cars in downtown Manhattan, where the authorities want you to begin your effort at problem-solving. When you arrive for your first day on the project, in downtown Manhattan in morning rush hour, you are surprised to find an almost deserted situation with fewer cars than one would expect even on the slowest New York day. You therefore conclude that the real problem is this lack of cars in downtown, and you order thousands of cars to be shifted from other areas of the city. Shortly after these cars arrive, a bottleneck on the cross-Bronx expressway clears up, an accident that has stopped traffic dead in the Lincoln Tunnel is finally cleared away, and the tens of thou sands of cars stuck on the periphery of the city come pouring into the now congested area that you have created by diverting other cars to downtown.

Obviously, your most serious error on this project, one that would doubtless cost you your job, was failing to ask for detailed maps not just of downtown Manhattan, but also of all of the tunnels and bridges and access routes coming from the other boroughs, New Jersey, and Connecticut. Without these maps as guides, you could not possibly understand the nature of the local congestion or lack of same in downtown Manhattan's traffic circulation. Congestion on the periphery of the city is clearly important for understanding the overall picture.

Well, I ventured with my students, many acupuncturists make the same error in their own work. They learn the local patterns of the ZangFu (downtown Manhattan) with very little understanding of the nature of the possible constrictions and dysfunctions in the various interconnected meridians and secondary vessels (the tunnels and bridges and access routes to 'downtown'). They therefore focus their attention on the local state of the internal ZangFu without the same attention to what has happened on the periphery: in the regular meridians, their internal pathways, and the union points between one meridian and another, where constrictions and congestion often occur, and the secondary vessels and the eight extraordinary vessels. Ignorant of this complex set of access routes, how could these acupuncturists ever hope to really understand the true nature of the congestion and dysfunction they find downtown, in the internal functions of the bodymind?

This question has concerned me for several years, and I am delighted that Matsumoto is bringing a new consciousness to the acupuncture community. Acupuncturists must know the stuff of acupuncture well— that is to say, the meridial access routes that lead into and out of the Sea of Qi inside the body. While a herbalist needs to focus his gaze to this internal Sea, an acupuncturist must be an expert in the periphery—access routes, tunnels, and bridges that service this Sea.

The Japanese concept of "Kori" studied by Matsumoto and Birch in *Hara Diagnosis: Reflections on the Sea*[1] says this all very well.

Kori refers to tense, constricted areas of the body, often manifested by pain, stiffness, and other subsidiary disturbances that result from this accumulation of tension. Kori is generally thought to be caused by a stressed lifestyle, poor diet, and lack of adequate exercise, leading to an accumulation of tension in the muscles. This tension in turn causes decreased oxygenation and flow of nutrients to the tissues, resulting in further contraction and tightening of the muscles, fascia, and connective tissues causing more pain and stiffness, etc. While acupuncturists all speak of "energy blockages," these can be seen more precisely, physiologically, to entail constriction in four systems of the body. The muscular tension of Kori constricts the lymph vessels, compromising the im.mune system; the venous system, resulting in buildup of wastes such as carbon dioxide and lactic acid with blood stasis; the arterial system, cutting down on oxygen and nutrients to the tissues; and the nervous system, leading to irritation, pain, and overly "facilitated" areas in which the nervous impulses misfire (akin to the concept in osteopathy of "trigger points"). These constrictions that compress the vital activities of these four systems thereby compromise the functions of the organs significantly. Acupuncturists in Japanese traditions who pay attention to these Kori areas, which can be found only through careful palpation, know that in releasing these constrictions they do not only alleviate pain and tension in the affected zones but also free up circulation in the lymph, venous, arterial, and nervous systems, improving overall regulation of the bodymind and enhancing immunity.

With patients who have Chronic Fatigue and Immune Dysfunction Syndrome, referred to in Chapter 6, those who take the time to palpate will find Kori to an impressive degree, with trigger points and muscular nodules so prominent in some cases as to warrant the diagnosis of fibromyalgia. Freeing up these tense areas leads to improved functioning throughout these patients' systems, with an increase in energy and stamina.

Matsumoto and Birch list the most common areas where Kori develops, which I have reorganized as follows (see the table on page 72) to show that they usually occur in the Yang meridians and zones, the big joints (areas where many divergent meridians begin), Chung Mo (part of the Yang Ming system, as we will see in Chapter 9) and the sternocleidomastoid (SCM) muscles of the neck, so crucial in autonomic activity according to Matsumoto's most recent studies.

Following are the points and zones that I palpate. Readers may also wish to consult the works of Kiiko Matsumoto for the various "palpation patterns" discovered by some Japanese practitioners who respect meridian energetics and believe, as I do, that the body speaks the language of energetics and that therapist and client alike can learn to read this somatic energetic language.

Greater Meridian Unit Tender Points

Taiyang	Shaoyang	Yangming	Chung Mo	Big Joints	SCM	Other
Bl. 10	G.B. 20 & 21	St. 11–12	Ki 11–21	Bl. 40	St. 9	Liv. 9
S.I. 11	T.H. 15	St. 21–30	St. 30–21	G.B. 34	L.I. 18	
Bl. 31–34	G.B. 27–30	L.I. 4 & 10	C.V. 2–14	St. 36	S.I. 16	
Bl. 54	T.H. 16	St. 36, 37, 39		Lu. 5		
Bl. 57–61	G.B. 31	Eyes of the knees		Per. 3		
Bl. 40	G.B. 34	From Taiyin = Lu. 1 & Sp. 16		Ht. 3		
Bl. 57	G.B. 37–38					

Greater Meridian Units—Three Levels of Being

Unit 1

Taiyin or Greater Yin (Lungs–Spleen): Sp. 1, 3, *4, 5,* 9, 10, *15, 20, 21; C.V. 12; Lu. 1,* 5, *7,* 8, *9.*
Yangming or Sunlight Yang (Large Intestine–Stomach): St. 43, 39, *37, 36, 30, 25,* 18, 12, 4, 3; L.I. *19–20,* 18, 11, *10,* 6, *4.*

Unit II

Shaoyin or Lesser Yin (Heart–Kidneys): Ht. *7,* 3, 1; Kid. *27, 23,* 21, 16, 11, *10,* 7, *3, 2,* 1; *C.V. 23, C.V. 6.*
Taiyang or Greater Yang (Small Intestine–Bladder): S.I. *3, 4,* 6, 7, 9, *10,* 11, *18;* Bl. *1, 10, 11, 12,* 54, 40, 58, 59, *64,* 67; *C.V. 3, 4.*

Unit III

Jueyin or Absolute Yin (Pericardium–Liver): Per. *6, 5,* 4, *1; C.V. 17, 18;* Liv. *3, 5,* 8, *9,* 13, *14; C.V. 10, 11.*
Shaoyang or Lesser Yang (Triple Heater–Gall Bladder): T.H. 3, *5,* 10, 15, *16, 22, 23;* G.B. *1, 3,* 13, 14, *20, 21, 22,* 24, 26, 29, 30, 31, 34,*40, 41,* 44.

Note: As shown above, the English translations for the Greater Meridian Units are as follows: Taiyin = Greater Yin; Yangming = Sunlight yang; Shaoyin = Lesser Yin; Taiyang = Greater Yang; Jueyin = Absolute Yin; Shaoyang = Lesser Yang. The *italicized* points are the key *points of union* where the two meridians—Lungs with Spleen; Large Intestine with Stomach for the first Unit—have energetic overlaps or places where their energy is most concentrated. The other points are also key points of each of the meridians. Thus, if I were palpating the Liver meridian, I would palpate all the points of the Liver channel under Jueyin above. But if I were palpating Jueyin as a Great Meridian unit, I would palpate the italicized points: Per. 6, 5, 1; C.V. 10, 11, 17, 18; Liver 3, 5, 9, 14. Palpation of both zones usually occurs for me simultaneously. If I initially suspect constriction in the Liver zone as a result of the intake interview, I will begin to palpate the Liver meridian (first on the left, as Matsumoto emphasizes) on both sides to see if one side is excess and the other is deficient, and then move to palpation of the Pericardium pathway on both sides. Often this will reveal upper left and lower right imbalance, or the reverse—for example, with excess in the Liver pathway on the leg on the left and of the Pericardium pathway on the left arm points, with deficiency of Jueyin, Liver and Pericardium pathways, on the right. Any of the various combinations of upper/lower and right/left are possible, and I check for these first.

ABDOMINAL STRESS REACTION PATTERNS

After observing abdominal palpation from Kiiko Matsumoto at a seminar at the Tri-State Institute several years ago, and trying it out with my clients for a year, I discussed with Kiiko the possibility of two common abdomens, a deficient yang of Spleen and Kidney abdomen, correlating with adrenal exhaustion and the parasympathetic stress patterns (ZangFu patterns of Earth, Metal, and Kidney Yang), and a constrained Liver Qi abdomen, correlating with sympathetic stress reaction patterns (the Kidney Yin, Wood, and Fire patterns of the ZangFu). She agreed, adding that about 80% of the population have one or the other abdomen, with 40% showing signs of one and 40% showing signs of the other. The remaining 20% of the population have a combination of the two, according to

FIGURE 6

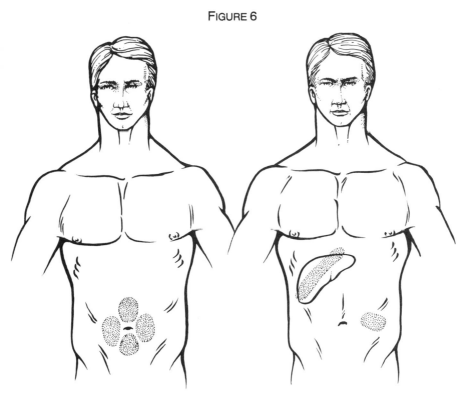

Left: *Abdomen of Fear and Exhaustion (parasympathetic dominant):* This constriction usually encompasses the duodenum, especially to the left of the navel, the duodenojejunal junction, and the adrenals, with repercussions throughout the small intestine and bladder.

Right: *Abdomen of Fight-or-Flight (sympathetic dominant):* This constriction usually encompasses the ascending colon and hepatic flexion of the colon, the liver and gallbladder, the transverse colon, and the lower aspect of the descending colon.

some Korean research which correlated these abdomens with sympathetic and parasympathetic system activity. I therefore always check for these two common Hara patterns, and teach my clients simple visualizing techniques and acupressure to focus their breathing on this Hara zone, thereby bringing their energetic center back down to the core in acupuncture-energetic terms. This often correlates, for me, with Eight Extraordinary Vessel treatment in a way different from the Japanese authors studied by Kiiko but consistent with their thinking and intention.

Also, I always palpate, where appropriate, the Mu and Shu points, with special attention in these days of immune deficiency to Bl. 14 and 43 (14 for panic syndromes and 43 for the immune system); Bl. 17 and 18 for the diaphragm; and Bl. 18, 20, and 23 for the immune system, as discussed in Chapter 6. This palpation is accompanied by statements appropriate to the imaging, as discussed above, and sets a clear context for the needling process.

COMMON VISCERAL CONSTRICTIONS REFLECTING ON THE HARA

In a workshop I attended with the prominent French osteopath Dr. Jean-Pierre Barral, author of *Visceral Manipulation* (Vols. 1 and 2), I was struck by the key sensitive areas he pointed out, referring to specific visceral constrictions, which invariably were points that I have come to focus on in my own practice, having found them to be congested very frequently in my clients. If Barral's theory of visceral constriction is correct— that once stressors invade the surface muscles and fascia, they are absorbed by the suspensory tissues, ligaments, and connective network that binds the viscera to the peritoneum, the diaphragm, or each other to maintain them in their proper place and motion— then the acupuncture release of appropriate points will free up these internal restrictions, making acupuncture a part of "visceral manipulation" in the strict bodywork sense of the word. Barral's theories should be read along with Matsumoto and Birch's *Hara Diagnosis*. Together, they promote an embodied view of acupuncture that focuses on the fascia, with the acupuncture points serving as entry points for our own type of body repatterning akin to Barral's bodywork.

Just as Matsumoto and Birch stressed that Kori (muscular tension) can build up in many areas of the abdomen, especially the subcostal regions, along the rectus abdominus muscles and linea alba, and in the region of the ASIS (anterior–superior iliac spine), the inguinal joint, and the superior aspect of the pubic bone, so too does Barral stress examining and freeing up these zones.

Specifically, we can see the following correlations between Barral's sensitive "visceral points" and acupuncture points: Liver 13 on the right relates to the lower right border of the liver and the hepatic flexure of the colon; Liver 14 on the right and left correlate with the suspensory ligaments of the liver; subcostal points like Kidney 21 and Stomach 21 relate to the liver and gallbladder on the right and the stomach and spleen on the left; Stomach 25 and Spleen 15 and 16 relate to the ascending colon on the right and the descending colon on the left; Gallbladder 27–28 relate on the right to the ileocecal valve and right ovary; Conception Vessel 2–3 relate to the bladder and Conception Vessel 4–6 to the lower aspect of the small intestine (as do the Kidney points of Chung Mo lateral to these C.V. points); Conception Vessel 9 –12 relate to the small intestine and pancreas; Kidney 18–20 relate, on the right, to the beginning of the duodenum and sphincter of Oddi, and, at Kidney 16 on the right, to the flexure from the second to the third part of the duodenum, with Kidney 18–20 on the left corresponding to the duodenojejunal junction; points near the xyphoid process, like Conception Vessel 14–15 and Kidney 21, relate to the transverse colon and to hepatic constrictions as they impinge on the pancreas and spleen [Chung Mo constriction in Hara diagnosis, or Liver (Gallbladder) invading Spleen-Pancreas (Stomach) in ZangFu acupuncture.]

Knowing what specific viscera these reflex points refer to, the acupuncture therapist can refine his focus to intervene more accurately on the connective tissues that serve as shock absorbers for the organs and bowels.

9

Clearing the Surface,
Supporting the Core

A CHOICE OF TREATMENT STRATEGIES

While I do have a general idea of treatment strategies (Mu/
Shu, Source/Luo, etc.) and precise points to select based on
my oral evaluation of the client, I finalize—and sometimes totally
revise—my choice of strategies and points only after careful
palpation as already explained. I expect, in other words, a
pattern of points to begin to *resonate* with the client and his
current condition, upon palpation. I expect a bodily felt
awareness to at least begin to emerge, a bodily "Ah Ha!"
experience that shows that the choice of pathways and points
makes sense as a start. In short, I expect the client to
acknowledge somatically that this is a relevant pattern of
points by his own confirmations: "What are those two points
related to!" or "How did you know exactly where to press?" or
"No, it's a little to the left." All of these responses indicate that
the person already knew which points needed to be prodded—
already was aware, that is, of his somatic-energetic patterns.
This realization grew out of my experience but found happy
confirmation in the groundbreaking work of Eugene Gendlin,
who developed the concept of *bodily felt sense* in psychotherapy, and Stanley Keleman, whose extensive experience in
bodywork led to a concept of somatic energetics and somatic

awareness very similar in many respects to my own. In his approach, which is by far the most developed presentation I have seen to date, there is a complex dynamic interplay between surface muscular defenses and inner bodily awareness. Taken together, the works of Gendlin and Keleman lead to a somatically grounded sense of body self and body-image, to complement and revive in a more pragmatic fashion Freud's original conception.

AN EMBODIED LIFE

Phenomenologists of the body, such as David Michael Levin with his concept of *body recollections,* and Eugene Gendlin with his concept of *bodily felt sense*, have succeeded in moving phenomenology one step further by grounding it (following Nietzsche and Heidegger) in the body, rather than in the sole realm of "consciousness." In this fashion, they mend the body/mind split and situate life's experiences within the felt realm as well as the conceptualized realm. Moving beyond Descartes' famous dictum "I think, therefore I am," they would state, "I think, from the conscious realm, and feel and sense, from the bodily realm, therefore I exist and give a shape as well as a meaning to my life."

Like these phenomenologists of the body, Stanley Keleman, a pioneer in modern bodywork and director of the Center for Energetic Studies in Berkeley, California, emphasizes that psychological understanding and insight are rarely sufficient to create change. "When we fail to understand our history as somatic organizations, we continue to repeat it," he says. "Emotional history, however, is a somatic organization which requires destructuring as well as reorganization."[1] In an utterly pragmatic yet decidedly phenomenological fashion, Keleman begins his work with people by focusing on the give and take of muscular contraction and elongation, seeing, as he does, that all sensations, emotions, and thoughts entail organized muscular somatic patterns and muscular waves.

In *Embodying Experience*, Keleman develops a straight-forward and highly useful clinical technique involving a five-step process for gaining somatic awareness of one's being, both in a particular situation or problem and in the larger context of one's life. Perceiving his work as behavioral educa-tion, he teaches clients how to intensify, then counter with opposite muscular patterning, their ways of holding their body in the space and time of their own unique life, so that they learn to recognize, from a bodily felt sense, their capacity for changing inappropriate or undesirable patterns. In doing this, they learn to trust a sixth, somatic sense, exactly as in Gendlin's work in psychotherapy. The body's way of posturing, constituting body-image and somatic images, can be con-sciously experienced, Keleman says, and therefore changed. In his perspective, we continuously create a variety of somatic shapes to meet internal and external stresses and strains of living. He educates clients to become aware, viscerally, of their own stress responses, first intensifying them in their body and then letting go, developing a countering relaxation response in order to prod the body to remember how to function more smoothly, relaxing a constricted zone of the body, firming up a sagging zone to shore up the spirit. This is decidedly similar to such Oriental practices as T'ai Chi Chuan or Qi Gong, where the interplay between form and no form in the first instance, and visceral awareness in the second, forms a core of Taoist practices for gaining control of one's bodily being in the world.

Through the physicality of his approach, Keleman enables clients to make tangible connections between the visible realm of outer actions and behavior and the invisible realm of inner sensations and feelings. "Our shape," he adds, "is a multilayered reality, each layer a structure of inner and outer reality."[2] Keleman divides these levels into three zones: genetic (prepersonal), societal (postpersonal), and personal. Together, these layers form our self as somatic image. "A somatic image is an anatomical or behavioral form. Skeletal muscles are responsible for posture, learned social roles, and instinctual gestures. They make a motif of sensations that give a body image, an external, somatic image. The pattern of visceral motility gives rise to sensations that establish an internal somatic image."[3] In this crucial reformulation of Freud's concept of body-image, Keleman emphasizes this dual nature of somatic awareness of self, with an inner aspect knowable only by oneself from the inside, and an external aspect facing toward the outside world and observable in one's body structure and behavior. "A somatic image, then, contains inner organ sensations and emotional configurations as well as body stances and action poses. A somatic image not only tells the world who you are, it also tells you who you are."[4]

As a phenomenologist, and like phenomenological psychologists,[5] Keleman emphasizes that we create our own space, our interior, our insides as bodily forms not given at birth, which some traditions might call soul or spirit. In this sense, then, we all create stories that shape our body-image. "A story is an experience of organized bodily responses. It involves muscular patterns of too much or too little form, too much or too little excitation."[6] Memory includes these muscular and excitatory patterns as our past history embodied in the present, according to Keleman. To change old behavioral patterns, then, it is not enough to remember intellectually or recollect emotionally. One must also revive the body's memory of a particular story, changing its muscular and excitatory patterns as well as its emotional and affective associations. Storytelling, a totally human practice, is an internal dialogue, in Keleman's view, that constitutes our body-image based on "the cellular feelings and the sensations of bones, muscles, and organs."[7] Every experience therefore entails form-making, *embodiment*, shape. In living our life, we give it shape, so that "we generate experiences and organize them into temporal configurations, the geometry by which the human, the personal and the universal is revealed."[8]

I have taken this long detour into Keleman's work because it articulates, based on much bodywork experience (bringing into play the work of Reich and bioenergetics, Alexander, and so on) the need to make inner and outer body-image connect. In my own work, I have come to see the need for connecting, energetically, with a person's *constitution* (Keleman's prepersonal), his *reactions to stress* (Keleman's societal, postpersonal), and his *present energetic state*, as a configuration entailing the other two realms. As I work with clients to guide them toward formulating their own energetic story, I often find it necessary to use metaphors that pertain to getting in touch with one's constitutional core or potential, and breaking down or undoing current somatic energetic reaction patterns that drain the bodymind and prevent access to deeper potentials, to reorganize the bodymind in such a way that change is possible. This behavioral, educational way of working came about by necessity, and it is gratifying and reassuring to see someone with as much clinical and educational experience as Keleman arrive at essentially the same place from a totally different starting point.

When acupuncture therapy is seen as part of this new Western body phenomenology (which itself is a reaction and complement to the one-sided self-psychology that has occupied Western attempts at self-awareness over the past one hundred years), new possibilities for working with our clients open up. As we cease to think of ourselves as healers, and instead perceive ourselves as educators or guides who help people *be their own healers,* we acupuncture therapists enter into an exciting dialogue that is currently engaging professionals, educators, and writers from behavioral and psychosomatic medicine, humanistic psychology, phenomenology, experiential forms of psychotherapy, and—more recently—orthodox medical and psychological practitioners. In this dialogue, we have much to offer and much to learn. As we go on to learn the Eastern practices of Chinese herbology, Qi Gong, massage, and so forth, we would do well to remain abreast of these other Western disciplines and the questions they raise. In this way, we will give shape to American forms of acupuncture therapy—as bodymind integrative practices—that embody our own efforts at understanding, from the energetic stories that we create as acupuncture therapists, how the psyche and the body process intercommunicate to give form to human existence.

A MULTI-LAYERED APPROACH TO ACUPUNCTURE THERAPY

In the following pages, the treatment strategies I most commonly use are listed in the order of preference I give them. I select these strategies in a way reminiscent of my early training in Van Nghi's three levels (Wei, Ying, Jing): in terms of treating on the level of *surface energetics, functional energetic* reaction patterns, or *core* or *constitutional energetics,* and adopt this three-part division to discuss those strategies I have come to rely on over ten years of acupuncture practice leading to a bodymind integrative perspective.

Surface Energetics

Conceiving of the energetics of the surface not only as the realm where Wei energy travels, according to tendino-muscular meridian theory, as the zone controlled by the Greater Yang Meridian Unit (Small Intestine and Bladder) in the Six Levels theory, and as the site of exogenous invasions of the atmospheric elements causing Bi (obstruction) patterns, but also as the bodymind's armor (or the external somatic image, to use Keleman's concept), we see that the simple act of needling into this surface is loaded with meanings and effects that go far beyond the skin and flesh.[9] The late Dr. Jean Schatz, past president of the International Society of Acupuncture and the European School of Acupuncture, emphasized the relationship between the surface-energetic realm of the tendino-muscular meridians and Wei energy, and Reich's character armor as described in his teachings.

Conceived in this fashion, intervention at the surface, to free up local obstructions by dispersing blockages, also puts therapist and client in touch with the core of the bodymind. It is therefore impossible, from this perspective, to free up the surface without touching larger issues of one's reactions to the outside world (except perhaps in some trauma cases). The reaction patterns carried out in the realm of surface energetics (entailing tendino-muscular meridian systems, trigger points, and Bi disorders) must be evaluated initially to determine whether the muscular-energetic zone is reacting in a specific way to an external stressor (for example, developing wandering spasms, twitches, and pains in the case of a "wind" disorder) as a unique, acute event, or whether this reaction is part of a series of responses by the bodymind always bringing into play the same meridian pathways or zones.

Disorders in this realm involve the skin, muscles, and

tendons (primarily in Yang, acute reaction patterns) or the joints (as is usually the case in Yin, chronic patterns of degeneration) and are therefore *insults to structure*.

If the disorder is a one-time, acute event, the only education required is to alert the client to the nature of the stressor (wind, cold, air conditioning, a fan blowing directly on the body during sleep, or repetitive stressful movements) so that he knows how to prevent a reccurrence. Treatment can then follow either the typical Bi syndrome treatment of TCM, treating painful or reactive local points with needles for wind or heat disorders, and with needles and moxa, or moxa alone, for cold or damp disorders, along with distal points that control the local area according to TCM strategies; or the tendino-muscular meridian strategies for excess and deficiency (Van Nghi, Low);or directly into trigger points.

For Excess of a Tendino-Muscular Meridian or Zone

Needle the local painful or reactive points rather superficially (I agree with Royston Low, and needle these points more deeply than Van Nghi's skin-deep insertion but less deep than in TCM Bi syndrome treatment, about 1/4 to 1/2"); pick distal points along the same tendino-muscular meridian pathways, selecting Jing-Well and Source points to marshall Wei energy into the tendino-muscular meridian(s) and to absorb exogenous pathogenic factors lodged in the meridian(s) and the tonification point of the corresponding regular meridian(s). According to Van Nghi, if the surface, Wei energetic realm is excess, the regular meridian level is relatively deficient and hence the need to tonify the deeper, regular meridian(s) to prevent a deeper penetration of the disorder. In disorders affecting the skin (contact dermatitis and so on), the musculature (spasms, strains, pulls), and the sinuses (sinusitis and rhinitis), including such disorders as TMJ syndrome and Bell's palsy, I find that tendino-muscular treatment is far more efficacious than Bi syndrome treatment, requiring fewer treatments with longer-lasting results. The key in this sort of disorder is careful palpation of the entire meridian(s) involved, as well as those in the same zone (tendino-muscular meridians all flow in groups—the Three Yang of the Hand; the Three Yang of the Foot; the Three Yin of the Hand; the Three Yin of the Foot). One must also treat the meeting zones (see Chapter 3 for the list of these points), often producing dramatic results.

For Deficiency of a Tendino-Muscular Meridian or Zone

Needle the local numb, weak, or reactive points superficially (possibly with gold needles), also using moxa or a heat lamp; needle the Jing-Well and Source points for the same reasons as above; needle the dispersal point of the corresponding regular meridian(s). According to Van Nghi, if the exogenous pathogenic factor manages to invade the surface and penetrates into the regular meridian level, Wei energy follows it, leaving the tendino-muscular surface-energetic realm deficient, with a subsequent excess in the regular meridian(s) due to the presence of the invading stressor and Wei as well as Ying (nourishing) energies. One must therefore disperse the regular meridian to rid it of the pathogenic factors. These conditions entail muscular atrophy and degeneration, joint diseases, and bone degeneration. Here it is also crucial to support the person constitutionally, for often the degeneration can only be slowed down, not reversed, and it is essential to shore up the core-energetic realm to prevent this skeletal or muscular degeneration from overly draining the energetic core, thereby affecting the spirit. In these degenerative conditions, I find that Bi syndrome treatment is often of equal value to tendino-muscular treatment. In these chronic, degenerative conditions, since they wear away at the integrity of the bodymind by sapping energy from the core, it is crucial to help clients be aware of the nature of the energetic breakdown so that they can behave so as to not exacerbate the situation, and it is also crucial to help clients try to get at the meaning of this degeneration. The life pressures, and one's ways of responding to them, must be understood by any client wishing to live productively with chronic pain or a degenerative condition of this sort, and the acupuncture therapist must therefore allow space for this dialogue (see Chapters 6 and 10, *Bodymind Energetics*). I find that these chronic surface-energetic conditions often occur along the Great Meridian Units, as in Requena's formulation. Thus, in addition to checking the Three Yang tendino-muscular meridian pathways of the Hand, for example, I will also check the Foot pathways of the same name (palpating all of Shaoyang, Taiyang, Yangming). For instance, a chronic tendino-muscular problem of the Triple Heater meridian, such as TMJ that affects the ears with accompanying tightness in the trapezius, will often coexist, or follow upon, a tendino-muscular holding pattern in the Gallbladder pathway as well, with tightness in the ribcage and hips, sciatica, and leg and foot pains that wander about (Gallbladder = Wood = Wind-like symptoms). Treatment of the entire Greater Meridian (Shaoyang, Lesser Yang in this case) is essential in such cases, and constitutes a truly etiological, rather than a merely symptomatic, treatment.

Functional Energetics

Once I have checked for, discounted, or successfully treated surface-energetic patterns, and at times concurrently with their treatment, I turn my focus to the functional-energetic realm of organ reaction patterns (ZangFu patterns). Conceiving of these patterns as behavioral reaction patterns, not as diseases or syndromes (as discussed in Chapter 5), and beginning with the most common stress reaction patterns involving the organ-energetic functions of TCM,[10] I work to help the client learn how he behaves, on the somatic-energetic level, in a day-to-day fashion, in such a way as to generate *insults to function*. Often having recourse to the classic psychosomatic concepts of organ or vegetative neurosis,[11] I reconceptualize the ZangFu patterns of TCM as common ways in which we all react viscerally to stress. After tending to any dysfunction in the stress reaction patterns (involving constrained Liver Qi and Liver Invading the Spleen, often with deficient Yang of the Spleen and Kidneys patterns, in TCM terms), including the Chung Mo and Kidney-Heart Protector anxiety and panic patterns,[12] I move on to focus with the client on target Organ-energetic areas, such as Spleen deficiency or Stomach excess, and work to help the client gain an awareness at the bodily felt level of how this function tends to break down. For example, does the Kidney Yang function begin to drop under the weight of sexual frustration or feelings of inadequacy with a new lover? Does the Spleen Qi function begin to sag under the weight of excessive worries and a life that does not nourish itself deeply, in the core of one's being? Does the Lung function begin to grow constricted at the constant loss of relationships, or grieving over the death of a loved one? These are the sorts of questions that arise in treatment of Organ-energetic functions as behavioral patterns that bring into play *constitutional* as well as *coping factors* (the way I reconceptualize what Worsley calls the Causative Factor, when speaking of the Elemental phases and the twelve Officials of traditional Chinese acupuncture). Here I often utilize the concept of the Officials as metaphors of vegetative function, in combination with the classic psychosomatic metaphors evoked above, in formulating a metaphor for the client. "Your Heart Protector function and Kidney-Fire seem to be deficient, making you too open to influences from the outside, which invade and drain you, with a subsequent loss of sexual passion and vitality, perhaps due to your high-pressured job, and all the unabated stress that goes along with it, as a medical social worker," I may state, to which the client may retort: "You've hit the nail right on the head. But these people need me; I am their only support; how can I find time to take care of myself in the face of such misery? What is my suffering compared to theirs? How can I close myself off to it?" As soon as such a metaphor fits, I shift into the client's metaphors and language. In this case, I would go with the images and ideas the client associates with needing to be "the only support" for so many people at the same time as refusing any nurturing himself, to help him see how his bodily responses of opening his Heart and chest too readily and subsequent loss of energy and sexual passion go along with this self-image. Often as the body image improves, as the protective barrier becomes more appropriate in this case for example, the self-image also improves, with an improvement in somatic as well as psychological functioning.

In these cases, I select treatment strategies from among TCM strategies of Local/Distal; Source/Luo; Mu/Shu (and often the second line of the Bladder meridian, for the Shen aspect of the Organ-function involved); Triple Heater regulatory points (Bl. 13, 15, 18, 20, 23 in combination, or C.V. 4, 6, 12, 17, 22); again using the Great Meridian Units to treat lower Absolute Yin (Jueyin, Liver) in disorders of the Upper Jueyin pathway (Heart Protector) for example, as I find that the Organ reaction patterns or target areas often bring into play an entire Greater Meridian Unit, as in Requena's work. I also often treat corresponding extra meridians to consolidate the effects of the

ZangFu treatments, seeing the extra meridians as the pre-organ realm, the realm of potential for all organ-energetic functions. The key, in these strategies, is the bodymind integrative approach one adopts with the client, seeing his problem as a behavioral one of adaptation and coping where he is brought into the center of the process and made to see his responsibility, and capacities, for change. This is very different from treatment of ZangFu problems as if they were objective diseases or disorders to be gotten rid of by the doctor.

Core, or Constitutional, Energetics

Once a person's musculoskeletal energetic defenses (tendino-muscular, surface energetics as character armor) have been tempered; and his stress responses and "organ inferiorities" (to quote Alfred Adler) have been alleviated or bolstered, energy is more available for focusing on the bodymind's energetic core, or constitution. The constitutional realm in acupuncture includes the Elements, stemming first from the Fire and Water Roots of the Kidneys, as predispositions that will affect all further organ-energetic functioning. A person with a deficiency in the Fire Root will grow cold, damp, and soggy, not only physically but emotionally. Conversely, a deficiency in the Water Root will lead to uncontrolled dryness and heat, general agitation, and emotional volatility.

It also includes the Eight Extraordinary Vessels, which appear first in the embryo and serve as the foundation, or core, around which the regular meridians, the secondary vessels, and the organ-energetic functions and structures develop throughout life. I use various ways of treating these vessels, stemming from French and Japanese traditions (see Low and Matsumoto). I also have a sense of the personality of each of these extra vessels and where they overlap with organ-functional patterns. Hence I treat Chung Mo where there is a predisposition to constrained Liver or Liver invading the Spleen, often with underlying deficiency of the Yang of the Spleen and Kidneys. I treat Ren Mo along with Yinchiaomo not only in those with fluid metabolism disorders, but also when the Lung-Kidney energetic vector is impaired (as in "Kidney asthma"). I treat Yinweimo alone, for persons whose Heart Protector function is impaired; with Chung Mo in eating and other gastrointestinal disorders of a truly psychosomatic nature, originating in infancy or adolescence; and with Kidney 2 and 3 and other Kidney Yang/adrenal regulatory points in panic and adrenal disorders.[13] For the Yang extra vessels, I treat Daimo in individuals whose character armor occupies the Shaoyang (Lesser Yang) zones, as Daimo is fed by the Gallbladder channel and brings together upper and lower, regulating the Three Heaters and the upper/lower polarities of the bodymind. I treat Du Mo along with Yangchiaomo in all people with stiffness of the spine and neck that accompanies a rigid or authoritarian personality structure, entailing the Bladder and Small Intestine Officials, as well as the Taiyang (Greater Yang) temperament as in Requena's work. Finally, I treat Yangweimo, along with Daimo, in people with Lesser Yang reaction patterns who hold their tension in their jaws and also have digestive disturbances (often Absolute Yin/Jueyin types, whose muscular patterns take the Yang corresponding pathways) and disturbed perspiration patterns.

While I find that character armor, as activated trigger points, usually develops along the Greater Yang Meridian Units (Shaoyang, Taiyang, Yangming), it is often as a coverup and protection for deficiencies or disturbance in the corresponding Yin functions. Hence, people with deficient Liver often have a hard, Lesser Yang protective cover. Freeing up the Gallbladder and Triple Heater Greater Meridian Unit usually is essential for supporting this constitutionally weak or chronically over-stressed Liver function. In treating the surface-energetic realm, as discussed in the chapter on palpation, I challenge the person to give up some of this tension, hoping that this will stir the deeper, core Organ-energetic function to accept energy from this released surface. In treating stress reaction patterns (the ZangFu, vegetative patterns of response) I become a behaviorist, helping the client localize target zones invaded by stress, and isolate the kinds of stress that set this pattern going. Finally, in treating core energetics, I encourage the client to construct a primal myth, an original metaphor that includes not only the first injuries to the bodymind function but the original source of bodymind strength as well.

SAMPLE TREATMENT PROTOCOL

What follows is the treatment protocol I teach my graduating students, as a sample of one style of practice. This is a good way to begin work with clients, in order to move from surface constrictions to deep energetic imbalances over a course of treatment. The following diagrams give the points for clearing the Greater Yang Meridian Units while at the same time supporting the Lesser Yin Units. The key dysfunctions for each zone are also noted.

I begin by assessing the constrictions (Kori) in TaiYang and Shaoyang, freeing up these zones in a way similar to Upledger's notions of cranio-sacral work. I palpate and de-activate the points of these two greater meridian units listed on page 73 and round out the treatment with the extraordinary vessel opening points for Du Mo, Yangchiaomo, Yangweimo, and Daimo (S.I. 3 and Bl. 62 for Taiyang; T.H. 5 and G.B. 41 for Shaoyang). After a few treatments, and once these zones are less tense and energy has been freed up to flow deeper,

I focus on tender points of Yangming, Chung Mo and Ren Mo, which serve as the shock absorbers for the front of the body (i.e., the rectus abdominus and linea alba as body armor). As outlined in Chapter 6, I treat sensitive points from Kidney 11–21 (Chung Mo); C.V. 2–13 (Ren Mo); Stomach 30 (Chung Mo and Yangming); from Stomach 29–21 (Yangming connected to Chung Mo, the two comprising the energetics of the rectus abdominus muscles); with distal points Sp. 4 and Per. 6 for Chung Mo and its paired Yinweimo; Kidney 2 and 3 for the Fire of the Kidneys (adrenal hyperactivity and exhaustion that usually ensues once stress is absorbed not only in the spinal Taiyang and lateral Shaoyang zones, but also in the ventral Yangming and Chung Mo/Ren Mo zones); Stomach 36, 37, and 39 (always with St. 25) for disorders affecting the small intestine, large intestine, etc., as are so common in Chronic Fatigue Syndrome, irritable bowel syndrome, functional hiatus hernia, and related disorders. I also check for the two common stress patterns related to deficiency below, excess above, namely Kidney Yang/Heart Protector imbalance (treating Kidney 2 and 3; Per. 4, 5, and 6; Bladder 14 and 43; and Bladder 23–25, and C.V. 6 and 9, Kidney 16 bilaterally and Kidney 22–23 with Per. 1); and Xu Li (treating Stomach 18 on the left, and C.V. 12, 17 and Stomach 12–16 where sensitive (on the left) with Stomach 43 or 42, or Stomach 40, where sensitive). These two patterns are reviewed in Chapter 6.

In these initial treatments, I focus on what I have come to view as the four phases of visceral agitation leading to visceral (and systemic) exhaustion, the most common stress patterns that I see (entailing disorders diagnosed as cervical syndrome, cervicalgia, brachialgia, lumbago, or craniosacral misalignment; irritable bowel syndrome; duodenal and ileocecal tension; various intestinal complaints; hiatus hernia and reflux esophagitis; gallbladder and liver congestion; pancreas dys-

DORSAL TREATMENT PROTOCOL

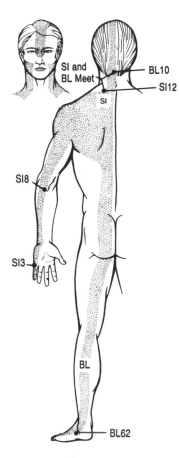

Dorsal: Greater Yang
(Small Intestine and Bladder)
Somatic Energetic Zones

Clearing Greater Yang:
Open key points;disperse
tender (trigger, Kori) points
throughout these zones.

Supporting Lesser Yin:
C.V.23 & Kid. 1; Kid. 2 & 3;
Heart 7 & 8; Bl. 15 & 23.

Extra Meridians in these Zones:
Du Mo, Yangchiaomo

Dysfunctions: stiff neck, tightness of the cervical region (where SI and BL meridians meet) and spine (SI3 governs the governing vessel); high blood pressure, constipation, diarrhea, Crohn's disease; urinary and prostate complaints; impotence, amenorrhea; Cushing's syndrome; ankylosing spondylarthritis; epilepsy, convulsions, vertigo, vertical occipital headaches, insomnia; psoriasis, eczema, acne on the forehead and upper back (SI and BL zones); paranoia, paranoid depressive states. Bladder Meridian "sciatica."

Key Points: SI3, BL62, SI12, BL10, plus local tender (trigger) points in the zones.

LATERAL TREATMENT PROTOCOL

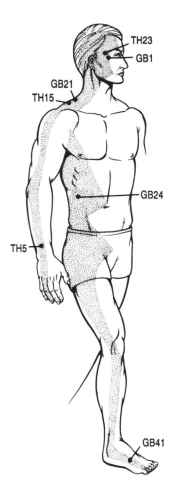

Lateral: Lesser Yang
(Gallbladder and Triple Heater)
Somatic Energetic Zones

Clearing Lesser Yang:
Open key points; disperse
tender (trigger, Kori) points
throughout these zones.

Supporting Absolute Yin:
C.V. 18 & Liver 1; Liver 2 & 3;
Per. 8 & 9; BL. 14 & 18.

Extra Meridians in these zones:
Dai Mo, Yangweimo

Dysfunctions: high blood pressure, stiff Belt Channel and lower back, difficulty rotating, varicose veins, phlebitis, stomach ulcers, constipation, hemorrhoids, arthritis (gouty), gall and kidney stones, facial muscle twitches or neuralgias, sweating disorders, clenched jaws, mandibular arthritis, arthritis of the hip joint, lateral sciatica.

Key Points: TH5, GB41, GB21, TH15, GB1, TH23, plus local tender (trigger) points in the zones.

VENTRAL TREATMENT PROTOCOL

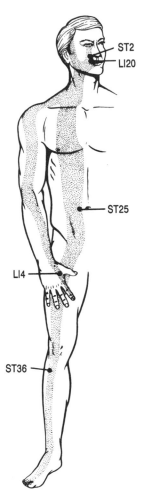

Ventral: Sunlight Yang
Stomach and Large Intestine)
Somatic Energetic Zones

Clearing Sunlight Yang:
Open key points;
open chung mo
(S.P. 4 & Per. 6 & Kid. 11–27
where tender); disperse
tender (trigger, Kori) points
throughout these zones.

Supporting Greater Yin:
C.V. 12 & Sp. 1; Sp. 2 & 3;
Lung 9 & 10; BL. 13 & 20

Extra Meridians in these zones:
Chung Mo, Ren Mo,
Yinweimo, Yinchiaomo

ST2
LI20
ST25
LI4
ST36

Dysfunctions: high blood pressure, cardiac disorders, mania, asthma, hiatus hernia, nausea, dyspepsia, vomiting, loss of appetite, colitis, constipation, hypothyroidism, shin splints, weakness, excessive hunger, eating disorders.

Key Points: ST36, L14, ST25, LI20, ST2, plus local tender (trigger) points in the zones.

function (including gastritis, pancreatitis; and hypoglycemia); cystitis, prostatitis, and other pelvic complaints; adrenal exhaustion with panic disorders, heart palpitations, or chest constriction, even asthma; mitral valve prolapse; fibromyalgia; and functional disorders of the thyroid. These stress disorders, so common and so well treated in acupuncture, often follow a movement from spinal irritations (phase 1) affecting the cervical or lumbosacral areas or both; to gastrointestinal irritation and agitation of the viscera there (phase 2); to pelvic irritation and agitation of the viscera there, with adrenal exhaustion (phase 3); to a "nervous heart" with agitation of the viscera of the chest, especially the heart protector (phase 4).

In acupuncture terms, we see a progression here from tendino-muscular and regular meridian constrictions in the meridians of Taiyang and Shaoyang, with perverse energy penetrating down Du Mo (phase 1). This is followed by penetration of perverse energy into Chung Mo, Ren Mo, and Yangming, often in the abdominal branches first (phase 2), followed or accompanied by penetration of perverse energy into the pelvic branches of these meridians (phase 3). Finally, when the root of the Kidneys is disturbed sufficiently by this struggle against perverse energy, with Kidney Yang deficiency (with excess Yin, water accumulation, etc.) or Kidney Yin deficiency (with hyperactive Kidney Yang), where Kidney Yang includes the adrenals, we have a disruption between the Lower and Upper Heaters, often with a totally constricted Middle Heater due to the chronic visceral irritation and exhaustion resulting from phases 2 and 3. This leads to Water not controlling Fire. All of these phases, taken together, occur in almost every case of Chronic Fatigue Syndrome I have treated, and acupuncture treatment as suggested above will prove extremely helpful with these complex cases.

After these treatments of phases 1–4, and sometimes

concurrently, I treat the three Yin—Taiyin, Shaoyin, and Jueyin—and the core, as outlined above.

In this way of working which Bob Flaws refers to as an "acupuncturist's acupuncture," I am always open to learning from my clients, and if a client comes up with an area or point that he feels needs to be treated, I usually comply, assuming as I do that I can do nothing more than prod the client's innate capacity to heal himself by prodding his will to be well. Knowing that I am not teaching my clients anything new, but rather am merely *imaging* their conditions in the bodymind-energetic terms of acupuncture energetics and psychosomatics, in order to catalyze their body's recollection of what it was given to know all along, I am never at a loss for new possibilities that may arise from the client's own innate knowledge. At every moment I have absolute faith in the client's ability to *change,* and I focus my work on that ability.

Appendix:
Self-Study Exercises

Following are some exercises that may be used by students, teachers, or practitioners of acupuncture, acupressure, shiatsu, jinshindo and other forms of bodywork based on acupuncture theories to move toward a meridian acupuncture (acupuncturist's acupuncture) perspective and way of working.

1. Take any of the patterns of disharmony of the ZangFu described in any TCM text, and try to correlate the signs and symptoms of the pattern with the meridians that flow through the affected zones. This will lead to a "meridians and secondary vessels" perspective of ZangFu disturbances, with further ways of intervening in these disturbances. While TCM acupuncturists focus on the ZangFu, it must be remembered that one always treats along meridians and at acupuncture points. A meridian perspective will therefore add depth to a TCM acupuncture practice and viewpoint.

2. Take the points given for any disorder (cystitis, for example) and draw them on a figure of the body. Then connect the dots to see what meridians are involved. In the case of disturbance of the bladder, in this example, one will see that the most commonly treated meridians are not the bladder meridian, but rather the three leg Yin channels which traverse and energize the bladder and its related structures.

3. When evaluating a client, try to palpate the meridians first, before asking any questions or doing the four exams, as described in Chapter 8. Write down your findings on a diagram of the body, and list the meridians that are constituted by these points. List whether the points/meridians are excess or deficient (as in Shiatsu). Then do a regular TCM diagnosis and see

how your palpation is confirmed by the four exams and eight principle evaluation. Note that it is perfectly viable to work as an acupuncturist by palpating in this fashion. Many Japanese practitioners such as Kiiko Matsumoto work in this way. Such palpation practice develops the type of insight and intuition necessary to practice an acupuncturist's acupuncture.

4. Take a partner or client, look at her or him, relax, and try to decide, without any talking or palpating, what meridians and points are most disturbed. Don't worry that this may be "nonsense." You may be surprised that you have a good sense of these imbalances very quickly. Many acupuncturists have an immediate "feel" of this sort, and can tell you in the first few minutes with a client what is imbalanced, tight, or tense. This knowledge is very much right-brained and comes in all at once, from many directions and through all the senses (including senses we don't even have words for). I find that, after five to eight years of practice, acupuncturists who focus on meridians develop these "extrasensory" powers of perception. I think we are all capable of this. TCM acupuncture, on the other hand, leads in the opposite direction, to analytical powers that often subjugate these sensory ones.

Endnotes

CHAPTER 1

1. First articulated in Mark D. Seem, with Joan Kaplan, *Bodymind Energetics: Toward a Dynamic Model of Health,* Healing Arts Press, Rochester, VT, 1987.

2. Seem and Kaplan, *Bodymind Energetics.*

3. Paul Unschuld, *New Medicine in China: A History of Ideas,* University of California Press, Berkeley, CA, pp. 54–58; Cf. also pp. 90–91; and Ted J. Kaptchuk, "Introduction," in *Fundamentals of Chinese Medicine,* N. Wiseman, A. Ellis, translators, Paradigm Publications, Brookline, MA, 1987.

4. Unschuld, *Medicine in China,* pp. 57–58.

5. Ibid., p. 58.

6. Ibid., pp. 251–261.

7. Ibid., p. 260.

8. Cf. Kiiko Matsumoto and Stephen Birch, *Five Elements and Ten Stems,* Redwing, Brookline, MA, 1985; and *Extraordinary Vessels,* Paradigm Publications, Brookline, MA, 1986; Royston Low, *Secondary Vessels of Acupuncture,* Thorson's Publishers, Limited, London, U.K., 1985; Yves Requena, *Terrains and Pathology in Acupuncture,* Vol. 1, Paradigm Publications, Brookline, MA, 1986; B. Flaws, C. Chace, M. Helme, *Timing and the Times—Chronicity in the American Practice of Oriental Medicine,* Blue Poppy Press, Boulder, CO, 1986; Mark D. Seem, *Acupuncture Energetics,* Healing Arts Press, Rochester, VT, 1987; Seem and Kaplan, *Bodymind Energetics;* Kaptchuk, "Introduction," in *Fundamentals of Chinese Medicine.* All these offer alternatives to the TCM approach.

9. *New Medicine in China,* pp. 54–55.

10. Cf. *Bodymind Energetics,* Chapters 1 and 11.

CHAPTER 2

1. I owe this concept of attention and intention to the teaching of Dr. Gerald Epstein, the founder of a phenomenological therapeutic practice informed by ancient Hebraic and Egyptian practices, which he terms "waking dream therapy" articulated in *Waking Dream Therapy: Dream Process as Imagination,* Human Sciences Press, New York, 1981.

2. C. Larre, J. Schatz, E. Rochat de la Vallee, *Survey of Traditional Chinese Medicine,*Traditional Acupuncture Foundation, Columbia, MD, 1982, p. 192.

CHAPTER 3

1. A. Chamfrault, N. Van Nghi, *L'Energetique humaine,* Charente Printers, Angouleme, France, 1969.

2. Low, *Secondary Vessels of Acupuncture.*

3. This discussion of the meridians draws on Larre et al., *Survey of Traditional Chinese Medicine,* Chapter 4.

4. Nguyen Van Nghi and Tran Viet Dzung, Recours Nguyen, translation of Vol. 1 of *Zhen Jiu Da Cheng,* Edition N.V.N., 1982, pp. 170–173.

5. Ibid.

6. As appears in Andre Faubert, *Trait Didactique d'Acupuncture Traditionnelle,* Guy Tredaniel Editions, Paris, 1977.

7. George Souli de Morant, *L'Acupuncture Chinoise,* Maloine, Paris, 1972, pp. 136–138.

8. Requena, *Terrains and Pathology in Acupuncture,* Vol. 1. Seem and Kaplan, *Bodymind Energetics,* Chapter 3.

CHAPTER 4

1. This chapter first appeared in slightly different form in the *American Journal of Acupuncture,* Vol. 14, No. 4, October–December 1986.

2. Flaws et al.,*Timing and the Times.*

3. Cf. *Journal of Traditional Chinese Medicine,* "Interview with Ted Kaptchuk, Peter Deadman, Giovanni Maciocia, and Felicity Moir," Vol. 20, 1986.

4. Cf. Matsumoto and Birch, *Five Elements and Ten Stems.*

5. Ted Kaptchuk's recent work to retrieve and rework the Oriental pharmacology knowledge of psychospiritual distress might well lead to a bodymind integrative herbal therapy better suited for such Western complaints.

6. Cf. Seem and Kaplan, *Bodymind Energetics.*

7. Matsumoto and Birch, *Extraordinary Vessels,* p. 247.

8. For a fascinating and provocative discussion of the Self and acupuncture in the West, see Caleb Gattegno, *Who Cares About Health? Educational Solutions,* University Press, New York, NY, 1979, pp. 140–143.

9. *Extraordinary Vessels,* p. 60.

CHAPTER 5

1. Cf. Seem, *Acupuncture Energetics.*

2. By far the best book on these ZangFu patterns is Jeremy Ross, *Zang Fu: The Organ Systems of Traditional Chinese Medicine,* Churchill Livingstone, New York, 1985. This text is the perfect book for Western students because it is a result of careful rethinking, by a Western practitioner, in a way that recognizes these ZangFu patterns as behavioral, does not ignore the preponderant role of the emotions, and sees the need for a careful schematic presentation. This is in marked contrast to *The Fundamentals of Chinese Medicine.* In the latter text, the translation group's concern for a standardized, literal translation leads to a turgid style that takes the soul out of TCM, rendering the patterns of the ZangFu as *unreal events* necessitating a made-up language. How could one hope to make a patient develop a real feeling for his "gastrosplenic Qi vacuity"; "center Qi fall"; "impaired depurative downbearing of lung Qi";

"counterflow ascent of stomach Qi"; or "brewing hepatocystic damp-heat!"

CHAPTER 6

1. Larre et al., *Survey of Traditional Chinese Medicine,* p. 124.

2. Ibid., p. 147.

3. Ibid., p. 128.

4. Ibid., pp. 128–129. See also the concept of visceral constriction and visceral spasms in Jean-Pierre Barral, *Visceral Manipulation* (Vols. I and II), Eastland Press, Seattle, 1988, 1989. Dr. Barral treats this deeper visceral defensive energy system.

5. Ibid., p. 192.

6. Ibid.

7. As quoted in Larre et al., *Survey of Traditional Chinese Medicine,* p. 175.

8. Cf. Larre et al., *Survey of Traditional Chinese Medicine,* pp. 171–172.

9. Cf. Larre et al., *Survey of Traditional Chinese Medicine,* p. 172.

10. Constrictions in these areas involve the suspensory tissues of the peritoneum and its contents, especially of the liver, gallbladder, duodenum, sphincter of Oddi, duodenojejunal junction, ileocecal valve, stomach, etc., according to Dr. Jean-Pierre Barral.

CHAPTER 7

1. For a detailed discussion of the client's will to be well as opposed to the will to remain ill, see Seem and Kaplan, *Bodymind Energetics,* Chapter 5.

2. This refers to the title of a provocative and far-reaching phenomenological treatise calling for a phenomenology of the body to complete the phenomenology of consciousness of prior phenomenologists: Michael David Levine, *The Body's Recollection*

of Being, Routledge and Kegan Paul, London, U.K., 1985.

3. Eugene Gendlin, *Focusing,* Bantam Books, New York, 1982.

CHAPTER 8

1. Matsumoto and Birch, *Hara Diagnosis: Reflections on the Sea,* Paradigm Publications, Brookline, MA, 1988, pp. 266–267.

CHAPTER 9

1. Stanley Keleman, *Embodying Experience: Forming a Personal Life,* Center Press, Berkeley, CA , 1987, p. 2.

2. Ibid., p. 38.

3. Ibid., p. 43.

4. Ibid., p. 45.

5. Cf. Seem and Kaplan, *Bodymind Energetics,* Chapter 4, for a discussion of phenomenological psychology and the exploration of inner space.

6. Keleman, *Embodying Experience*, pp. 51–52.

7. Ibid., p. 52.

8. Ibid., p. 88.

9. Cf. Seem and Kaplan, *Bodymind Energetics*, Chapter 6 (skin), and Chapter 10 (musculoskeletal system), from a bodymind-energetic perspective.

10. Cf. Chapters 5 and 6.

11. Cf. Seem and Kaplan, *Bodymind Energetics,* Chapters 4–10.

12. Cf. Chapter 6.

13. Cf. Chapter 6.

Index

ACUPUNCTURE ENERGETICS
A Workbook for Diagnostics and Treatment
Mark D. Seem, Ph.D., Dipl. Ac. (NCCA)
ISBN 0-89281-435-7 144 pages, 5 1/4 x 8 1/2, $10.95

The first educational textbook on acupuncture designed for Western students and practitioners, *Acupuncture Energetics* offers an innovative approach to diagnosis and treatment planning in acupuncture that integrates Eight-Principle and Five-Phase diagnosis. A workbook section, keyed to major texts widely used in the field, includes case studies and self-study exercises, and provides an excellent resource for those who are preparing for licensure examinations.

"While the concept of Acupuncture Energetics breaks completely new ground, the author's simple and direct approach is in line with pure Traditional Chinese Medicine. This highly original book deserves a place in the curriculum of all schools of acupuncture."
–Royston Low, Ph. D., Dr. Ac., Past President, British Acupuncture Association

ACUPUNCTURE TREATMENT OF PAIN
Leon Chaitow, D.O., N.D.
ISBN 0-89281-383-0, 192 pages, 8 x 10, $16.95

Dr. Chaitow presents a method of effective pain control for use by those in the healing professions — acupuncturists, surgeons, general practitioners, osteopaths, chiropractors, physiotherapists, and trained nurses — as an adjunct to their normal course of therapy. Includes a formulary for pain treatment and shows the use of acupuncture as anesthesia and its use in the treatment of addictions.

"...tears away much of the mystique of acupuncture to present a simple approach to pain relief."—**The American Journal of Acupuncture**

ACUPRESSURE TECHNIQUES
A Self-Help Guide
Julian Kenyon, M.D.
ISBN 0-89281-280-X, 5 1/4 x 8 1/2, $8.95

Especially written for home use, this fully illustrated guide shows how finger and thumb pressure can be safely applied over specific acupuncture points to effectively treat a wide range of disorders, including sports injuries. Dr. Kenyon is past chairman of the British Medical Acupuncture Society.

BODYMIND ENERGETICS
Toward a Dynamic Model of Health
Mark D. Seem, Ph.D., Dipl. Ac. (NCCA), with Joan Kaplan
ISBN 0-89281-246-X, 288 pages, 6 x 9, $14.95

Through an integration of the principles of Traditional Chinese Medicine and psychosomatics, author Mark Seem moves beyond the existing medical models to develop a new energetic paradigm of health care — one that acknowledges the spirit of the individual seeking treatment as well as the fundamental connections between energy, body, and mind.

"Mark Seem's remarkable and innovative work explores new possibilities, using acupuncture to inform psychology and modern psychosomatics to expand contemporary acupuncture practices. This dialogue will not only enrich the two participant medical systems but will also contribute to the entire field of health, medicine, and healing."
–Ted Kaptchuk, Author of *The Web That Has No Weaver*

AMMA
The Ancient Art of Oriental Healing
Tina Sohn, as told to Donna Finando
ISBN 0-89281-229-X, 8 1/2 x 11, $14.95

Practically unknown in the West, Amma therapy dates back 5,000 years in China, and is the forerunner of all modern Oriental bodywork. This finely illustrated book is the first to detail the techniques of one of the few living masters of this ancient healing art.

"Reveals, for the first time, methods of achieving and maintaining health, validated not merely by evanescent modern science but by centuries of theoretical development and pragmatic application." **—Robert S. Mendelsohn, M.D.**

These and other Inner Traditions/Healing Arts Press titles are available at many fine bookstores or, to order direct, send a check or money order for the total amount, payable to Inner Traditions, plus $2.00 shipping and handling for the first book and $1.00 for each additional book to:

Inner Traditions/AIDC
64 Depot Road
Colchester, VT 05446
1-800-445-6638 (outside Vermont)   878-0315 (within Vermont)
Be sure to request a free catalog.